Zohra Dhouibi
Amine Trabelsi

Superfoods

Zohra Dhouibi
Amine Trabelsi

Superfoods

ScienciaScripts

Imprint

Any brand names and product names mentioned in this book are subject to trademark, brand or patent protection and are trademarks or registered trademarks of their respective holders. The use of brand names, product names, common names, trade names, product descriptions etc. even without a particular marking in this work is in no way to be construed to mean that such names may be regarded as unrestricted in respect of trademark and brand protection legislation and could thus be used by anyone.

Cover image: www.ingimage.com

This book is a translation from the original published under ISBN 978-620-6-70445-4.

Publisher:
Sciencia Scripts
is a trademark of
Dodo Books Indian Ocean Ltd. and OmniScriptum S.R.L publishing group

120 High Road, East Finchley, London, N2 9ED, United Kingdom
Str. Armeneasca 28/1, office 1, Chisinau MD-2012, Republic of Moldova, Europe
Printed at: see last page
ISBN: 978-620-8-19720-9

CONTENTS

1   *INTRODUCTION* *2*

2   *GENERAL DEFINITION* *3*

3   *MICRO-ALGAE* *6*

4   *LES LEVURES* *16*

5   *THE SEEDS* *31*

6   *THE LEAVES* *44*

7   *MACA ROOTS* *62*

8   *RED FRUIT* *71*

1 INTRODUCTION

In today's society, food is seen as a means of improving quality of life and fighting disease. There is a growing public interest in healthy foods that not only provide essential nutrients, but also boost the body's functionality and help prevent various health problems.

Superfoods" is a concept that emerged at the beginning of the 20th century when people started to take an interest in eating well. At the time, the focus was on foodstuffs that were the heroes of the plate, rich in nutrients and offering consumers the luxury of responding to the need to improve their own health, in line with the culture of homemade food [1]. They are also known as functional foods which, in addition to their nutritional functions, contribute to the proper functioning of the body, by presenting properties that are beneficial to health and/or reducing the risk of disease.

Superfoods, as described by Hanni Rützler, a nutritionist specialising in food trends, represent an age-old human quest that we're desperate to embark on, especially when it comes to foods of exotic origin. Brazilian acai berries, goji berries and spirulina powder, for example, are well integrated into this approach [2].

With growing consumer interest in healthy eating, superfoods represent a fast-growing commercial sector: the global market for functional foods was valued at USD 129 billion in 2015. This market is growing steadily year on year [1].

In this book, we will attempt to define the concept of 'superfoods' and determine their place in today's society, as well as detailing the monographs of certain foodstuffs considered to be superfoods and verifying their various uses and interests.

2 GENERAL DEFINITION

Although the concept of superfoods is of great interest to contemporary society, there is no relevant, standardised definition or classification of these foods. For the moment, there is no standardised or technical definition of the term "superfood". Rather, it is a fashionable expression that is essentially used as a marketing concept to promote and advertise the foods concerned. Most of these foods are rich in vitamins, active metabolites or enzymes. Superfoods are marketed in various forms, including as food supplements or as dried or fresh foods [2]. Superfoods" are generally exotic products that are little-known or unknown. They are part of the popular culture of a country or the folklore of a people or nation, which in short reveals the ethnography of eating habits. Superfoods are therefore usually used in the traditions of indigenous societies, such as berries, roots or seeds, and most often come from faraway regions. However, local foods such as blueberries, beetroot, avocados, salmon, herbs and spices are increasingly being considered as superfoods. Superfoods are now making their way onto supermarket shelves, whereas in the past they were marketed specifically in specialist health food shops and boutiques. A wide variety of superfood products are also being produced and marketed. These include pure chia seeds and flax seeds, as well as crunchy muesli, crusty bread and cereal bars with seeds. The list of superfoods is long and endless, and is revised and updated every year. Even dieticians are unable to give these foods an official, scientific definition. Dieticians are still sceptical about superfoods. It's true that there have been a number of studies showing the beneficial effects of a particular foodstuff, but most of these studies have been carried out on animals or in vitro, using isolated cultures of human cells. There is no certainty as to the effects that can be observed on human beings, particularly in the context of everyday life.

David Wolfe, an American food expert, talks about superfoods as being halfway between medicinal plants and food. In fact, in a world of consumerism, the aim is to provide consumers with simple, accessible solutions. As a result, simple statements such as "these berries work against disease" get a lot of attention, and of course the consumption that goes with it. The use of smoothies or berries and seeds as healthy, fast-absorbing ingredients, rich in numerous substances that promise to heal, or the administration of capsules that guarantee well-being, seem to respond adequately to our society's need for ready-to-eat foods. According to Neon magazine: "Smoothies are well suited to our times. They combine ancestral wisdom (fruit and vegetables are good for you), new technologies (cold pressing) and time efficiency (you can drink them quickly between two meetings)". A sort of combination between practicality and health, satisfying consumers' current desire for science and romance, which makes superfoods remarkable products. Nevertheless, there are misleading nutritional and health claims, where the qualities touted on packaging are far removed from those put forward in books on superfoods. The health claim made to the European Union (EU) for acai has been withdrawn. Similarly, the European Food Safety Authority has not authorised advertisements extolling the health benefits of goji berries. In addition, health claims for chia seeds are no longer tolerated, although it is permitted to say that chia seeds contain valuable protein and are a good source of alpha-linolenic acid (ALA) combined with a high level of dietary fibre. Otherwise, claims about the components of a product are authorised, but not the product itself. According to C. Daeniker of the Federation of Migros Cooperatives, by law no one has the right to say that food X has an effect Y on health. However, it is perfectly legal and fair to talk, for example, about the benefits of proteins and their necessary role in maintaining muscle mass and contributing to normal bone density [2].

Regardless of the criticisms of the fashionable term "superfood", it makes perfect sense to encourage the search for and identification of health-promoting components in natural foods, while at the same time suggesting replacement products that already exist in our country and not simply responding to the demands of a growing market for a new trendy food. Let's not forget that what is described as a 'superfood' today will be replaced tomorrow by another allegedly miraculous new product [2].

3 MICRO-ALGAE

3.1 Spirulina

3.1.1 Description

Spirulina occurs naturally as a symbiotic, filamentous, multicellular blue-green micro-algae. It uses nitrogen from the air and takes the form of a spiral or disc-shaped stem. The blue colour of this algae is due to phycocyanin, the main photosynthetic pigment in spirulina. It grows naturally in alkaline and warm environments, in the sea and in freshwater in subtropical and tropical regions, including Central Africa, Europe, Asia, America and Mexico [4].

It is officially known as *Arthrospira* (*Spirulina*), from the *Oscillateriaceae* family, belonging to the cyanobacteria class. In nature, the spirulina genus contains several species. Three of these species are being studied in particular, because they are edible and have significant nutritional potential and therapeutic value. These three species are *Spirulina platensis* (*Arthrospira platensis*), *Spirulina maxima* (*Arthrospira maxima*) and *Spirulina fusiformis* (*Arthrospira fusiformis*) [6].

3.1.2 History

Initially, spirulina was studied for its nutritional value as a food source. Over 400 years ago, spirulina was consumed as food by the Mayas, Toltecs and Kanembus in Mexico during the Aztec civilisation. In Mexico, *S. maxima* was usually abundant in Lake Texcoco. It was used in pre-Hispanic times to prepare a meal called *"Tecuitlatl"*. Later, during the Spanish conquest, it was harvested, dried and sold for human consumption. Spirulina harvested from Lake Kossorom (Chad) has also been consumed by Central Africans for centuries in the form of broths [7].

In the mid-70s, the intergovernmental organisation IIMSAM "*The Intergovernmental Institution For The Use Of Micro-Algae Spirulina Against Malnutrition*" was launched. Its aim was to promote spirulina as a highly nutritious food to combat malnutrition and famine on a global scale, due to its exceptional nutritional value [7]. Spirulina is currently considered a nutraceutical food supplement. In fact, the *National Aeronautics and Space Administration* (NASA) and the *European Space Agency* (ESA) have recommended spirulina as one of the main foods for long-term space missions, due to its high nutritional value [8].

The different species of spirulina and the products derived from them are used in pharmaceuticals, agriculture, perfumery, food processing and medicine. In Japan, spirulina has been marketed in tablet form since 1975. Spirulina is also used as an additive in foods (bread, biscuits, noodles, etc.) to boost their nutritional value. Phycocyanin is also used as a colouring agent in the food industry (sweets, drinks, health foods, etc.), the cosmetics industry and the pharmaceutical industry [9].

3.1.3 Composition

The composition of spirulina may vary depending on the growing conditions and analysis methods used. The composition of spirulina is **shown in Table I** which shows the results obtained by a third-party laboratory and by *Earthrise Nutritionals LLC* (CA, USA).

Table I: Nutritional profile of spirulina powder (composition per 100 g) [7].

Macronutrients	Vitamins

Calories	373	Vitamin A (in the	352,000
Total fat(g)	4.3	form of β-carotene)	IU
Saturated fatty acids	1.95	Vitamin K	1090
Polyunsaturated fatty acids(PUFAs)	1.93	Thiamine HCL	µg
Monounsaturated fatty acids	0.26	(vitamin B1)	0.5 mg
Cholesterol	<	Rivoflavin (vitamin	4.53
Total carbohydrates (g)	0.1	B2)	mg
Dietary fibre	17.8	Niacin (Vitamin B3)	14.9
Sugars	7.7	Vitamin B6	mg
Lactose	1.3	Vitamin B12	0.96
Essential amino acids (mg)	<		mg
Histidine	0.1	**Minerals**	162 µg
Isoleucine		Calcium	468 mg
Leucine	1000	Iron	87.4
Lysine	3500	Phosphorus	mg
Methionine	5380	Iodine	961 mg
Phenylalanine	2960	Magnesium	142 µg
Threonine	1170	Zinc	319 mg
Tryptophan	2750	Selenium	1.45
Valine	2860	Cooper	mg
Non-essential amino acids (mg)	1090	Manganese	25.5 µg
Alanine	3940	Chrome	0.47
Arginine		Potassium	mg
Aspartic acid	4590	Sodium	3.26
Cystine	4310		mg
Glutamic acid	5990	**Phytonutrients**	<400
Glycine	590		µg
Proline	9130		1,660
Serine	3130		mg
Tyrosine	2380		641 mg
	2760	Phycocyanin (average)	17.2%
	2500	Chlorophyll (average)	1.2%
		Superoxide dismutase	531,000
		Gamma linolenic acid	1080
		(GLA)	UI
		Total carotenoids	504 mg
		(average)	211 mg
		Beta-carotene	101 mg
		(average)	
		Zeaxanthin	

The vast majority of plant-based foods, even those known to be a good source of protein, contain no more than 35% protein. Spirulina stands out for its exceptional protein content, which is between 60 and 70% of its dry weight. In fact, one of the main proteins present in spirulina, accounting for around 20% of its dry weight, is phycocyanin-C. This is a water-soluble protein. This molecule contains phycocyanobilin, a biliverdin homologue [7]. As well as the exceptional presence of proteins in spirulina in terms of quantity, it is also important to note their quality. In fact, spirulina contains all the essential amino acids in a very high proportion, accounting for almost half of all proteins [10].

The lipid fraction in spirulina is present in a proportion of around 4 to 10% of its dry weight and is of significant value as it is a good source of gamma-linolenic acid (GLA), linoleic acid (LA) and oleic acid. Spirulina has the capacity to accumulate 1% of its dry weight in GLA. In addition, the concentration of decosahexaenoic *acid* (DHA) in *S. platensis* can reach 9.1% of its total fatty acids, making it an important natural source of DHA [7]. Spirulina is a good source of vitamins because it is rich in beta-carotenes and vitamin B12. One kilogram of spirulina contains around 700-1700mg of beta-carotenes, which are converted in the body into vitamin A. This vitamin is important for the proper functioning of the human body, and is required at a rate of 1mg/day. You only need to consume 1 to 2g of spirulina daily to cover these requirements. Finally, spirulina's high vitamin B12 content makes it a good alternative for vegetarians [7]. We are mainly interested in calcium, iron and phosphorus, which are the inorganic nutrients present in spirulina in the most relevant proportions in relation to the other minerals. In fact, plant-based foods contain only non-heme iron, the absorption of which is more likely to be altered by absorption inhibitors [7].

3.1.4 Therapeutic properties

The antioxidant and anti-inflammatory properties of phycocyanin, a component of spirulina, were first highlighted in 1998, and have since been confirmed by numerous studies [8]. A clinical study evaluating the effect of spirulina on aspirin-induced ulcers reported favourable results, highlighting spirulina's antioxidant and anti-inflammatory effects [11]. In addition to vitamins C and E, which are well-known non-enzymatic antioxidants, spirulina is rich in phenolic acids, beta-carotenes, GLA, selenium and certain amino acids such as cysteine and methionine [11].

Due to its tissue-protecting antioxidant properties, spirulina inhibits carcinogenesis and also reduces liver and kidney toxicity. Spirulina could be effective against diseases caused by free radicals [7,8]. Spirulina may also play a role in cardiovascular disease (CVD) through its antioxidant, anti-inflammatory and lipid-lowering properties [8]. A study on *S. platensis* concentrate suggests that the active component of spirulina responsible for the lipid-lowering effect is phycocyanin. Spirulina also acts by correcting the carbohydrate and lipid profile in diabetic patients and laboratory animals. It therefore plays a role in the metabolic regulation of lipids and carbohydrates. In the light of recent studies, it has been discovered that spirulina may exert a protective effect in metabolic syndrome and obesity. In a clinical study, it was reported for the first time that spirulina could have a promising anti-obesity potential and could be used, as a dietary supplement, to modify the mineral status of obese hypertensives receiving conventional antihypertensive treatment. This slimming effect was also highlighted in another study conducted in Germany [7].

With regard to vitamin supplementation, a clinical trial has shown that spirulina supplementation can correct vitamin A deficiency in children diagnosed with vitamin A deficiency. On the other hand, spirulina supplementation for children suffering from macrocytic anaemia showed no improvement in the anaemia. At present, knowledge of the mechanisms of activity of the various effects of spirulina is still limited. More in-depth studies are needed to identify its active ingredients and elucidate its therapeutic mechanisms of action [8].

3.1.5 Safety/toxicity profile

The long history of consumption in Mexico and Central Africa shows that spirulina can be considered safe for human consumption. This has also been confirmed in several animal studies. However, few clinical studies have systematically confirmed this notion in humans [8].

Nevertheless, the safety of consuming spirulina has been called into question following reports of some side effects. In fact, spirulina grown in open water sources has been found to contain low concentrations of heavy metals. Such spirulina preparations can cause heavy metal poisoning, particularly from mercury. Controlling the water sources used to grow spirulina means that mercury and lead concentrations are well below the standards set by the Food and Agriculture Organisation (FAO) of the World Health Organisation (WHO).

In addition, a recently published study showed that certain species of cyanobacteria are capable of producing a cyanotoxin called anatoxin-a. Anatoxin-a was found to be acutely neurotoxic in 3 of the 39 cyanobacteria samples tested. Contamination of spirulina products by such species of cyanobacteria can present a danger to consumers. Hence the recommendation for quality control of food supplements derived from cyanobacteria to avoid possible adverse effects in humans [8].

Finally, there have been rare reports of side-effects following spirulina consumption in humans, which should be taken into consideration: one case of hepatotoxicity, another case of rhabdomyolysis and an immune system disorder in a healthy 82-year-old woman, which manifested as bullous pemphigoid and pemphigus foliaceum [8].

3.2 Chlorella

3.2.1 Description

Chlorella is a cosmopolitan freshwater taxon. It belongs to the kingdom of chlorophytes *(Chlorophyta)* which have photosynthetic activity [13]. It is a unicellular microalga in coccoid form (<10μm) and its habitat is freshwater. *Chlorella vulgaris Beijerinck* has been established as the type species and more than 100 species of *Chlorella* have been described, most of them of freshwater origin. Due to incomplete descriptions, many of these species have been classified in a section of doubtful species, which has made it possible to reduce the number of *Chlorella* species [14].

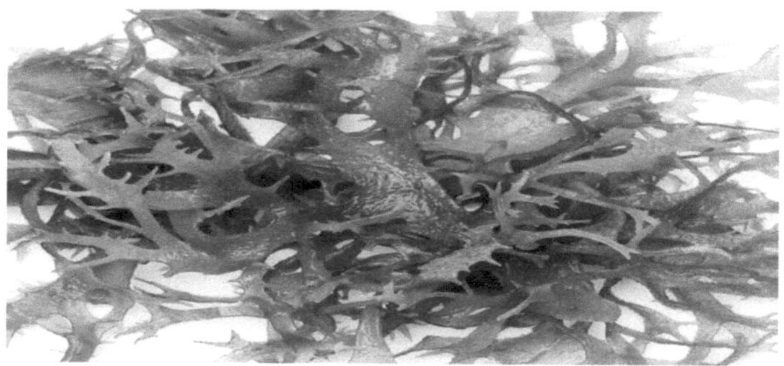

Figure 1: Chlorella [15]

Generally speaking, spherical green species, mainly freshwater or terrestrial organisms, are considered to belong to the genus *Chlorella*. Some phylogenetic studies have shown that *chlorella* is a polyphyletic organism belonging to different classes [14]. In fact, the study of the taxonomy of the genus *Chlorella* is a process that is still under review. *Chlorella salina* is one of the first described species of the genus *Chlorella*, and is distinguished from *Chlorella vulgaris* only by its presence in the marine environment. These two species have morphological similarities. Other marine species include *Chlorella spaerckii* described by Alvik, *Chlorella capsulata* described by Guillard et al and those described by Butcher: *Chlorella marina, Chlorella ovalis, Chlorella salina, Chlorella stigmatophora* [14].

3.2.2 History

The *Chlorella* genus was the first microalgae to be massively cultivated for human and animal consumption. It is a well-known and popular food, particularly in Asian countries such as Japan, Taiwan and Korea [16]. More than 70 companies worldwide produce *C. vulgaris*. It is currently marketed in Asia as a nutritional supplement. It was initially produced in the form of algal biomass or extract by the food industry. Subsequently, the biomass has been used to produce a variety of health products such as tablets, capsules, powder or for the extraction of bioactive ingredients. Algal extracts are used as food enrichers or additives to improve the nutritional and health value of various common foods, mainly liquid foods such as soft drinks, tea or beer [9].

3.2.3 Composition

Chlorella contains proteins, minerals, vitamins, dietary fibre and a wide range of antioxidants, bioactive substances and chlorophylls. This microalgae is an important source of PUFAs, proteins and phosphates. Due to its richness in lutein, zeaxanthin and beta-carotene, *Chlorella* is considered a good dietary source of carotenoids for humans [9]. It has also been shown that it is necessary to process *C. vulgaris* to ensure sufficient bioaccessibility of the carotenoids. In addition, a study has shown that *C. vulgaris* is richer in pigments, particularly carotenoids and chlorophylls, than *S. platensis* [17]. Chlorella is widely known for its ability to store energy. According to a Korean study, *C. vulgaris* is rich in important PUFAs such as ALA (45.8%, 50.8mg/g) and hexadecatrienoic acid (11.8%, 13.1%). As a result, this microalga could have potential as an important source of PUFAs [18].

3.2.4 Therapeutic properties

Due to its high nutritional profile, *Chlorella* appears to be a promising raw material for the formulation of functional foods. Indeed, chlorella has shown significant pharmacological properties in several studies, not only in animal models but also in human clinical trials. According to Okudo et al, consumption of chlorella in patients with hypercholesterolaemia reduces their blood cholesterol levels [19]. Fujiwara et al. have also shown that eating chlorella has a beneficial effect on hyperlipaemia. This property was also demonstrated in another study where daily supplementation with *Chlorella* in subjects with mild hypercholesterolaemia effectively reduced cardiovascular risk factors linked to serum lipids, mainly triglycerides (TG) and total cholesterol. This effect is mainly linked to carotenoids [16].

In addition, Nakamura et al. proved that *C. vulgaris* intake reduced blood pressure in hypertensive individuals. In addition, supplementation with chlorella for 6 weeks in male smokers had a positive effect on their antioxidant profiles. In fact, it has been reported that, in vivo, the carotenoids contained in this microalga have positive effects on antioxidant status and serum lipid risk factors [16].

On the other hand, one study has suggested that short-term supplementation with chlorella has a beneficial immunostimulant effect in normal healthy individuals, by improving the activity of *Natural Killer* (NK) cells and the early inflammatory response [16]. Thanks to its high β-glucan content, *C. vulgaris* has antitumour, immunomodulatory and hypoglycaemic properties. It has anti-metastatic activity thanks to the glycoproteins it contains [19]. *C. vulgaris* has been shown to reduce inflammation and improve glycaemia and liver function [20]. One study clearly showed that enzymatic hydrolysates of chlorella have high digestibility values as a sustainable and reliable protein source. Consequently, conventional sources in nutraceutical formulations such as soy, whey and fish proteins could be replaced by hydrolysates from these microalgae. In addition, an animal study showed that a *Chlorella-based* diet induced weight gain and protein bioavailability ranging from 58% to 77% apparent biological value, and that fat absorption was lower than for soya oil in a control diet. *C. vulgaris* could therefore be used as an alternative source of protein and omega-3[21].

3.2.5 Safety profile/Toxicity

Chlorella has been a safe and well-tolerated source of human nutrition for centuries [19]. According to the classification of the Centre for Food Safety and Applied Nutrition, microalgae biomass is classified as an 'other food supplement'. *Chlorella* is classified by the *Food and Drug Administration* (FDA) as a "Generally *Recognised As Safe*" (GRAS) food source [22].

An experimental study evaluating the safety of *C. vulgaris* showed that chlorella supplementation at different doses in mice over a period of 14 days had no adverse or toxicological effects. No cardiac, hepatic or renal toxicity appeared in histological or serum analyses following diets based on this microalga. Diets rich in *Chlorella* are therefore well tolerated, well accepted and adequate to ensure proper organ function and maintain body weight [23]. However, an experiment involving an animal tumour model suggested that *C. vulgaris* administered at a high dose (200mg/Kg) could promote tumour growth. Such hypotheses should be explored by in-depth studies in the future [24].

4 THE LEVURES

4.1 Red yeast rice

4.1.1 Description

Also known as *Monascus purpureus* rice, red yeast rice (RYR) is derived from the *M.purpureus Went* yeast strain and is prepared using a traditional rice fermentation method [25]. LRR fermentation uses micro-organisms that are various species of a filamentous fungus known as *Monascus* [26]. Monascus spp belongs to the *Aspergillaceae* family, genus *Monascus* [27]. The mould belongs to the polyketid family and is mildly bactericidal. The Monascus group includes *Monascu.anka*, *Monascus.ruber* and a strain of *Monascus.ruber* known as *Monascus.purpureus* (*ruber* and *purpureus* are the Latin words for red and purple, respectively). These fungi are capable of producing an intense red pigment and other metabolites when grown on cooked non-glutinous rice [26,28].

Following fermentation, the product obtained is in the form of scarlet to violet grains that retain the structure of the original rice grain (**Figure 4**). In China, this fermentate is known as "*Ang Khak*" or "*Hong Qu*". It is also known in Japan as "*Koji*", "*Ang-Khak*", "*Beni-Koji*" and "*Red-Koji*". It is also known as "*Rotschimmelreis*" in Europe and "*Red Mold*" in the United States [29].

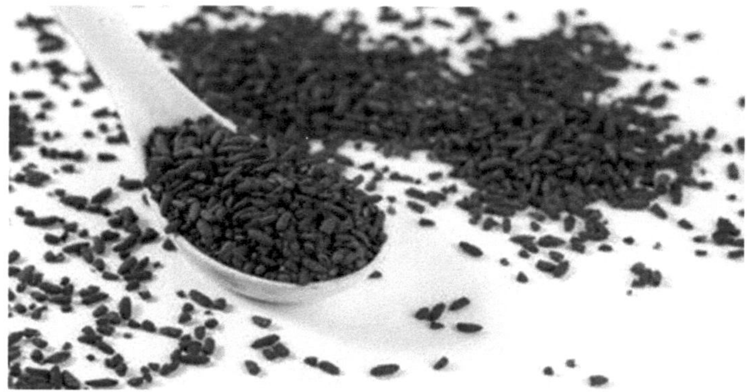

Figure 2: Red yeast rice [30]

Regarding the strong colour of *Monsacus* fermentate, yellow, red and orange pigments are responsible for this coloration. These pigments are secondary metabolites of *Monascus* fermentation. They belong to the group of azaphilones, which are typical fungal metabolites. Depending on the presence or absence of the yellow or red pigments and their predominance, the colours of *M.purpureus* vary from yellow-orange to scarlet-red to purple-red. The production of a specific colour pigment can be controlled by modifying the substrates, the fermentation conditions (temperature, pH, dissolved oxygen, the source of phosphorus, carbon and nitrogen) and the fermentation mode (solid-state or submerged fermentation) [25].

4.1.2 History

PBR was first described more than 2,000 years ago in the monograph by Li- Shin-Chun (1590). This book describes the usefulness of the LRR pigment as a food colouring, preservative, flavouring and therapeutic agent for treating various diseases [31]. In East Asian countries, solid-state fermentation of rice by *Monascus* has a long and ancient tradition dating back to at least the first century AD [32]. In Asia and Indonesia, the products of rice fermentation, such as PBA, have been consumed for centuries as staple foods and food additives. The use of LRR is well known in Japan, China, Taiwan, Okinawa and the Philippines for preserving meat and fish, for adding colour and flavour to foods, and even for brewing wine and alcohol. In addition, an ancient Chinese pharmacopoeia of medicinal foods and herbs, Li Shi-zhen's *"Ben Cao Gang Mu"*, mentions that PBA can be effective as a medicine for revitalising the blood and improving digestion [33]. For centuries, *M. purpureus* rice has been used as a food supplement and herbal medicine in China [25]. In Japan, *Monascus* extract is marketed as a dietary product (under the name Monacolin by Maruzen) [28]. PBA is marketed in capsule form with a dosage of 1.2 to 2.4 g/day, corresponding to 5 to 10 mg of monacolin per day, in divided doses for a trial period of up to 3 months [33, 34]. PRA is currently used in the food industry in several Asian countries as a food additive, particularly as a condiment and meat preservative. Thanks to its high alpha-amylase content, which promotes the conversion of starch into glucose, LRR is used to make rice wine. Monascus pigments give rice wine its attractive red colour. Generally speaking, meat products containing *Monascus* extract are considered to taste better than comparable products without *Monascus*. In fact, during fermentation, rice proteins are partially hydrolysed by *Monascus* enzymes, releasing the oligopeptides responsible for the *Monascus* flavour effect [25].

4.1.3 Composition

M.purpureus produces natural pigments. All pigments are chemically stable. More than 90 different molecules can be produced by *Monascus*, but only six pigments are known and they come in three colours. These are a group of orange pigments called monascorubine and mubropunctatine, yellow pigments called monascine and ankaflavine and red pigments called monascorubramine and rubropunctamine [35]. These pigments can be used as an alternative to the certified food colours or natural pigments currently in use. As well as being used to colour meat, fish, cheese, pâtés and beer, these natural pigments are also used in the textile, cosmetics and pharmaceutical industries [36].

In addition to rice starch, protein, fibre, trace elements such as magnesium, sterols, unsaturated fatty acids (oleic, AL, GLA) and B-complex vitamins such as niacin, PRA contains several active substances, including monacolin K, dihydromonacolin and monacolin I to VI. PBA is a staple food in Asia and was quickly recognised in the United States as a cholesterol-lowering agent [25, 26, 33].

4.1.4 Therapeutic properties

Monascus fermented products and their secondary metabolites have received a great deal of attention over the last few decades, due to their therapeutic effects on a variety of ailments. Secondary metabolites include isoflavones, enzymes, fatty acids, organic acids, dimerumic acid (antioxidant), vitamins, gamma-aminobutyric acid (hypotensive agent) and monacolin K (lovastatin, anti-hypercholesterolaemic agent) [1].

LRR has been shown in animal and clinical studies to be effective in reducing serum lipid levels. In fact, some LRR compounds inhibit HMG-CoA reductase, which is responsible for inhibiting cholesterol synthesis in the liver [25]. PBA can be used to treat hyperlipidaemia. PRA extract helps to lower cholesterol levels, reduce LDL levels, increase HDL levels and lower TG levels. It does all this by inhibiting hepatic production of cholesterol itself. This action is due to mevinoline, also known as monacolin K, a compound chemically identical to lovastatin, which is sold as a cholesterol-lowering drug [33, 37]. Mevinoline also has a structure similar to the active ingredients in cholesterol-lowering drugs such as simvastatin and atorvastatin. In parallel with the animal trials carried out to assess the LRR, it has been studied as a treatment in certain human trials. Daily administration of 1.2g (approximately 5 mg total monacolins) of LRR to men and women for two months showed significant reductions in serum cholesterol levels [34]. In addition, there was an increase in HDL cholesterol associated with a decrease in LDL cholesterol and TG levels in the serum of people consuming LRR. Similar results have also been shown in other studies using PBA as a dietary supplement [33, 34]. A recent meta-analysis highlights the efficacy of relatively safe PBA for dyslipidaemia, which may be an alternative approach in patients with a history of statin-related adverse effects and could also be used to prevent coronary heart disease. Nevertheless, there is a lack of sufficient evidence and rigorously designed, long-term randomised studies to recommend PRA to patients with dyslipidaemia, particularly as an alternative to statins. Similarly, further trials of PBA in patients with CVD, diabetes and other diseases associated with dyslipidaemia are warranted [38].

In addition to monacolins, PRA contains many other synergistic nutrients with lipid-lowering activities, including sterols such as beta-sitosterol and campesterol, which interfere with cholesterol absorption in the intestines [33]. In fact, the combination of these dietary sterols with statins has been suggested as a more effective cholesterol-lowering treatment than statins alone [39]. PRA PUFAs in turn reduce serum lipid levels [34].

Scientific research has confirmed that *Monascus* fermentate has a preservative effect. In fact, one of the compounds isolated from *M.purpureus* cultures, called monascidin A, has an inhibitory effect on bacteria of the *Bacillus*, *Streptococcus* and *Pseudomonas* genera. In addition, it has been shown that two of the yellow pigments in *M.purpureus*, when used in low concentrations, have a bacteriostatic action against *Bacillus subtilis* [28]. Similarly, an inhibitory effect has been observed, particularly against *Staphylococcus aureus*. The bacteriostatic effect of *Monascus* fermentate has been evaluated in further research, where it was found that Gram-positive bacteria (BGP) are generally more strongly inhibited than Gram-negative bacteria (BGN), while *Lactobacillus* are unaffected. The bacteriostatic properties of *Monascus* fermentate have led to it being considered as a substitute for nitrite for preserving meat [1].

In addition to protecting against CVD, a Chinese study showed that PRA extract also had the advantage of increasing insulin sensitivity and lowering blood sugar levels in a group of type 2 diabetics (T2DM). In the light of other studies, it has been suggested that LRR may have other interesting applications, such as the use of lovastatin and other statins in the treatment or prevention of cancer, osteoporosis, atherosclerosis, stroke, Alzheimer's and other dementias and macular degeneration [1, 40-42].

4.1.5 Safety profile/Toxicity

As research and applications have become increasingly focused on *Monascus* and its metabolites, concerns about its potential toxicity and safe consumption have also grown [1]. LRR is generally well tolerated. Nevertheless, it may have some temporary adverse effects such as burning of the intestinal tract, dizziness and bloating [34]. In addition, this product is contraindicated in people suffering from liver disorders. Some side effects have been reported following consumption of PBA, including headaches, gas, digestive discomfort and dizziness. Such effects are generally mild and resolve quickly when the drug is stopped. A risk of rare but serious reactions may occur with 'statins' in PBA extract, including skeletal muscle damage, liver damage and kidney toxicity. Such reactions also occur in 1% to 2% of people taking the drug lovastatin and may include unexplained weakness, muscle pain and tenderness and other flu-like symptoms. However, a 12-week clinical trial of LRR extract showed that kidney and liver function remained normal [40, 42]. In addition, another study showed that LRR is a safe and effective cholesterol-lowering agent in the treatment of nephrotic dyslipidaemia in children and adults [43].

In addition, *Monascus* produces citrinin, which is the dominant mycotoxin in this species. Citrinin has been identified in commercial samples of *Monascus* at levels of 0.2 to 1.71 µg/g. This mycotoxin is capable of damaging liver, kidney and body tissues and has been assessed as a carcinogen. In fact, there is a relationship between citrinin production and toxicity and the strain, environment, temperature and nitrogen and carbon concentration. To avoid toxicity and safety problems, a maximum dose of citrinine is set in LRR-based food supplements. This dose is around 200 ng/g in Japan, while it is 2mg/Kg in the EU [1].

While the *European Food Safety Authority* (EFSA) approves and encourages the use of monacolin K extracted from LRR (at least 10mg) for the treatment of hypercholesterolaemia [44], the FDA considers monacolin K to be an unapproved foodstuff, due to its similarity to lovastatin, and subsequently prohibits the marketing of products containing a specific amount of monacolin [45]. PRA should always be used with caution, and is not recommended for pregnant or breastfeeding women, those being treated with other cholesterol-lowering drugs at the same time, or those with a serious infection, organ transplant or major surgery. In addition, it is important not to drink more than 2 alcoholic beverages a day and not to consume large quantities of grapefruit juice while taking PRA. In sufficiently high doses, it can cause muscle pain and fatigue. It is therefore important to implement an incremental dosage schedule, at least initially [25]. It is advisable to provide LRR-based products with the necessary warnings, since they expose patients clinically to the same potential risks as statins [46].

Future studies are needed to discover other ways of experimenting with lower levels of potentially toxic compounds and optimising fermentation processes to produce high-quality secondary metabolites that are more effective in therapeutic and food applications [1].

4.2 Brewer's yeast

4.2.1 Description

Yeasts are a heterogeneous group of highly important micro-organisms that are currently attracting increasing attention from scientists and industry. The genus Saccharomyce is the most extensively studied of the yeasts belonging to the phylum *Ascomycota* [47]. It is a genus of ascomycetous yeast characterised by round to oval multilateral budding yeast cells with the presence of short, rudimentary *pseudohyphae* (sometimes well developed) [48]. *Saccharomyces cerevisiae* (**Figure 5**) is one of the best-known yeast species in terms of health and well-being. It is more commonly known as brewer's yeast (B.L.) or baker's yeast [49]. The *S.cerevisiae* species is very heterogeneous, with several strains belonging to this species with specific capacities, such as sherry wine strains, *S.boulardii* or baker's yeast strains [50]. Most of the dry weight of the yeast cell wall is made up of polysaccharides which form the skeletal framework defining the stability of the cell wall and cell morphology (beta-D-glucans) [51].

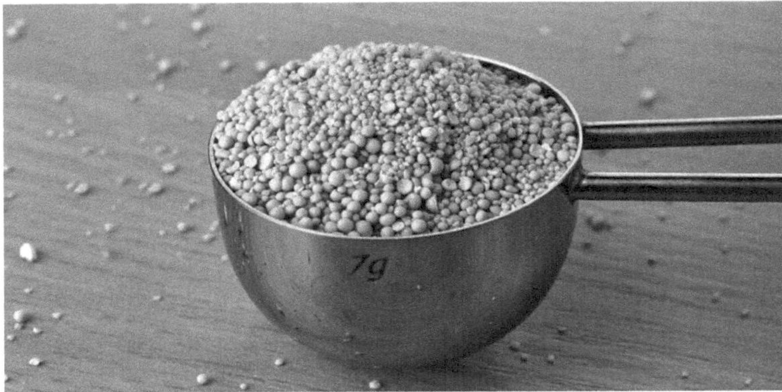

Figure 3 Brewer's yeast [52]

In nature, yeast cells are found in fluctuating environments where they are often subjected to food shortages. For example, oak bark, one of LB's natural habitats, subjects it to seasonal cycles of tree sap flow, in addition to climatic conditions. *S.cerevisiae* cells are therefore most of the time in a state of non-division called quiescence [53]. Yeasts have relatively simple nutritional requirements [47]. Under favourable conditions, *S.cerevisiae* can grow on a modest range of fermentable and non-fermentable carbon sources. Primarily, they use carbohydrates as a carbon source, essentially hexose sugars in the form of monosaccharides (glucose, fructose, galactose or mannose) or disaccharides (maltose or sucrose) [54]. The growth programmes and rates as well as the behaviour of yeast cells can be directed by the availability of key nutrients, such as sugars, amino acids and nitrogen compounds. In response to their nutritional environment, these cells are able to adjust their behaviour and modify the length of their cycle. They can range from rapid mitotic growth in rich environments, to filamentous growth in limiting conditions, to various distinct resting states, each allowing survival under conditions of particular nutrient deprivation [55]. Thanks to our ability to control and manipulate the life cycle of *S.cerevisiae* it has become the most powerful unicellular eukaryotic system for biological research and has been rapidly adopted worldwide for practical studies of all aspects of biology [56].

4.2.2 History

Fermentation is one of the world's oldest methods of processing and preserving food. Since ancient times, yeasts and their metabolic products have been exploited by humans primarily for baking and brewing. Today, modern yeast biotechnology products have become indispensable in many important commercial sectors, including food, beverages, pharmaceuticals, LB-based dietary supplements, industrial enzymes and others. *S.cerevisiae* has been exploited by humans for over ten thousand years for brewing and baking. Industrial *S.cerevisiae* yeast strains, including baker's, wine, brewer's and distiller's strains, show significant heterogeneity and present multigenic families [57].

Due to applications such as alcoholic fermentation, bread-making, single-cell protein production, vitamin production and recombinant protein synthesis, several species belonging to the *Saccharomyces* genus are of great biotechnological importance [47].

Nowadays, there are several products derived from yeast fermentation, including yeast cells and yeast extracts. These products are known to improve appetite and fibre digestibility and inhibit pathogen growth. LB is also used as a protein supplement, energy booster, immune enhancer or other vehicle where other compounds can be inserted to create a marketed health product [49]. For example, the design of a food supplement enriched by the use of *S. cerevisiae* yeast as a cholecalciferol accumulator [58]. One of the most notable positive results came from a large randomised trial in which adults were given a modified LB-based product (EpiCor) on a daily basis after having recently been vaccinated against seasonal flu in order to prevent colds and flu symptoms. The LB product significantly reduced the incidence and duration of this common condition [49].

4.2.3 Composition

LB contains several functional ingredients, it is a rich source of fibre (mainly β-glucans), protein (including proteolytic enzymes), vitamins and minerals. *S.cerevisiae* is an important source of vitamin B2 and mainly vitamin B1. The recommended daily intake of vitamins B1 and B2 is found in 5g of yeast. To identify LB, the ratio of vitamin B1 to B2 is used as a criterion. Generally, LB has a ratio greater than 1. However, a vitamin B1 content of 4 mg per 100 g or more, combined with a vitamin B1 and B2 ratio greater than 3, indicates good quality LB [59]. The use of β-glucans from *Saccharomyces*, known as yeast β-glucans, as an ingredient has already been approved by EFSA, which suggests consuming between 50 and 200 mg per portion [60]. Yeast proteins and proteolytic enzymes are considered to be GRAS, while presenting an adequate amino acid profile rich in essential amino acids, with sulphur amino acids at levels above the FAO/WHO reference [61, 62]. Thanks to its economic impact, *S.cerevisiae* is probably the most important species in its genus. It is the yeast most commonly used in food fermentation. Annually, *S.cerevisiae* is used to produce around 60 million tonnes of beer, 30 million tonnes of wine, 800,000 tonnes of unicellular proteins and 600,000 tonnes of baker's yeast [63]. The European yeast industry produces 1 million tonnes each year, with around 30% exported worldwide. From 2013 to 2018, the annual growth rate of the global yeast market was 8.8% [64].

4.2.4 Therapeutic properties

S.cerevisiae has a number of beneficial effects on human health and well-being, of which the probiotic effect is the best known [51]. While the development of foods containing probiotic compounds has focused mainly on *Lactobacillus* and *Bifidobacterium*, the yeast *S.cerevisiae var. boulardii* has long been known as a treatment for gastroenteritis [47]. It was first identified in 1984 from lychee fruit in Indonesia, and studied for its potential use as a probiotic. It subsequently became a probiotic species intended for human consumption, the efficacy of which has been documented in numerous clinical trials. To date, only the *S.boulardii* strain is considered to be a probiotic yeast, as more definitive in vitro characterisations of other 'alternative' species need to be established before they can be used in human trials and applications [65]. It is, in fact, the only yeast that is used and produced as a pharmaceutical product offering several valuable effects such as immunomodulatory effects and the prevention and treatment of intestinal diseases in children and adults as shown in several studies. In addition, it has been shown to reduce antibiotic-associated diarrhoea in hospitalised patients [66, 67]. In addition, yeast cell wall polysaccharides, notably known as β-glucans, are water-insoluble and non-digestible and may modulate mucosal immunity of the intestinal tract, facilitate intestinal motility and be used in constipation, among other intestinal problems [68]. *S.cerevisiae* yeasts have widely known antagonistic activities towards undesirable bacteria and fungi. Such activities are related to their competitiveness for nutrients, the acidification of their growth medium, their tolerance to high concentrations of ethanol, and the release of antibacterial compounds and antimicrobial compounds such as antifungal killer toxins or mycocins. The latter were first identified in the brewing industry [47]. *S.ceravisiae* also has other beneficial therapeutic effects, such as lowering serum cholesterol. In one study, evaluation of the effect of daily *S.boulardii* supplementation on cholesterol in hypercholesterolaemic adults for 8 weeks showed a reduction in residual lipoprotein, which is a predictive biomarker and potential therapeutic target in the treatment and prevention of coronary heart disease [69]. In addition, the β-glucans constituting the yeast cell wall possess immunomodulatory properties and are therefore applied in anti-infectious and anti-tumour therapy [51]. On the basis of several clinical trials presented in a review, it has been shown that an increased intake of β-glucans can stimulate the immune system. This has been confirmed by a large body of research into the immunomodulatory effects of yeast β-glucans [70]. Recent data have also suggested that polysaccharides isolated from the baker's yeast S.cerevisiae have an antioxidant effect and therefore protective potential as antioxidants, antimutagens and antigenotoxins and may be involved in cancer prevention and therapy [51]. Because of its glucose tolerance factor, a recent study has shown that dietary LB supplementation combined with the usual treatment of T2DM in diabetic patients can have beneficial effects on insulin receptors and can therefore improve glycaemic variables in these patients [71]. It may also reduce systolic and diastolic blood pressure in T2DM patients [72]. LB is also consumed as a nutritional supplement to boost vitamin intake and is mainly recommended for pregnant and breastfeeding women, people recovering from illness and growing children [73].

4.2.5 Safety profile/Toxicity

In general, LB-based products are very well tolerated [70]. In addition to its high nutritional value, *S.cerevisiae* has a high fermentation capacity with a lower toxic potential [74]. According to EFSA, *S.cerevisiae* has QPS ("*Qualified Presumption of Safety*") status [75]. Although *S.cerevisiae* baker's yeast has a long history of safe consumption, rare allergies can occur following its consumption in food [76].

Dietary intake of β-glucans isolated from LB has been shown to be very well tolerated in all clinical trials. No signs of toxicity have been reported. Their safety may be related to their mode of action [70]. However, it has been reported in some publications that parenteral β-glucans have adverse toxicological effects such as hepatosplenomegaly and granuloma formation. Such events have never been reported after oral application [77]. An EFSA scientific opinion considered that the allergenic risk of yeast β-glucans is no higher than that of other baker's yeast products [78]. Although invasive infections caused by *S.cerevisiae* are rare, a first case of osteomyelitis caused by *S.cerevisiaea* was reported in a post-traumatic patient. The outcome was favourable after surgical debridement, prolonged antifungal treatment and hyperbaric oxygen therapy [79]. Furthermore, an analysis of a total of 51 samples of LB from the German market revealed natural contamination of 63% of these samples by ochratoxin (OTA). These results suggest a potential risk of ingesting OTA by consuming food supplements based on natural LB from the brewing process. Hence the recommendation to screen LB food supplements for OTA as part of food safety and quality control [73].

Single-dose acute and sub-chronic animal toxicity studies in rats showed no signs of toxicity from *S.cerevisiae*. Neither deaths nor abnormalities were caused by single doses of 2000 mg/Kg. In addition, oral administration for 91 days at 100 mg/Kg body weight showed no adverse effects or toxicity in rats [80]. Furthermore, it has been suggested in several studies and analyses of the potential virulence of *S.cerevisiae* species in vivo and in vitro that certain strains have the potential to cause disease irrespective of their origin of clinical or non-clinical isolation [81, 82]. Indeed, animal studies on different strains isolated in clinical environments and from a dietary supplement have shown that there are strains with a very low level of virulence and others with a relatively high level of virulence [83]. Opportunistic strains of *S.cerevisiae* have thus been defined as those that have the physiological characteristics of yeast pathogens, such as growth at 37°C, but can also cause infections and kill mice, unlike most other strains [82, 84].

Compared with other micro-organisms such as viruses, bacteria and certain filamentous fungi, yeasts, particularly *S.cerevisiae*, have an impeccable food record. Large viable populations of *S.cerevisiae* are consumed by humans without their knowledge or care, and without any adverse effects on their health (for example, yeast in home-brewed beer, yeast-enriched beers or the yeast-containing food supplements that are very common today). But you still need to keep an open mind and be vigilant about yeast and dietary diseases. Yeasts are not considered aggressive pathogens compared to other microbial groups, however, they are capable of causing human illness in opportunistic circumstances [57]. Based on the progress of research into the nature of the virulence mechanism of *S.cerevisiae* strains, greater attention should be paid in the future to industrial practices that are more likely to generate opportunistic strains of *S.cerevisiae* [**50**].

5 THE SEEDS

5.1 Soya beans

5.1.1 Description

Soya (*Glycine max (L.) Merrill*) is one of the world's most important crops, ranking sixth with production of 347 million metric tonnes in 2017-2018 **[85]**. *Glycine max* (**Figure 6**) belongs to the Fabaceae family. It is native to Asia. The United States, Brazil, Argentina, China and India are the world's soybean producers, with global production volumes of 35%, 28%, 17%, 4% and 3%, respectively. Italy is the European country with the highest soya production, with 933,140 tonnes per year **[86]**.

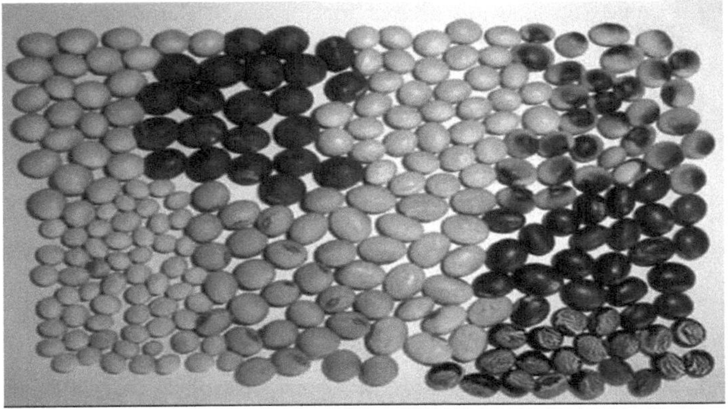

Figure 4: Soya beans [87]

The colour of the soya bean coat is an important characteristic that determines the external appearance of the soya bean.   The   colours range from yellow, green, brown and black to two-tone **[88]**. Black soya has been used in traditional medicine in China, India, Japan and Korea for hundreds of years. The size of soybeans and their isoflavone content vary according to climatic conditions and cultivation practices [89].

5.1.2 History

Historically, the main consumers of soy have been identified in Asian populations, this is due to many traditional Asian foods using soy as the main ingredient. Nevertheless, the consumption of soya-based foods in Western countries has increased over the last decade with the trend towards a vegetarian lifestyle and a healthy perception of soya consumption [90]. As a result, a wide variety of soy-based food products are available in grocery shops. In addition to market demand, the popularity of this product is linked to the nutritional and versatile properties of soya beans, which are suitable for technological food processing. Soybeans have the advantage of being used to produce several analogues and substitutes for meat and dairy products which could be used as alternatives, particularly when following a vegetarian diet [91]. For example, in the UK, the main soya-based foods consumed are soya-based dairy substitutes, and soya 'meat' is very popular in Denmark [92]. Soy oligosaccharides have also been proposed as substitutes for prebiotics or sugars [93]. Soya is traditionally used in Asian regions to prepare a number of dishes. Mixing and heating soya beans produces soya milk, which can also be treated with $MgCl2$ or curdled $CaSo4$ to produce tofu. It is also useful to carry out several fermentation processes to obtain natto, tempeh, soy sauce and sufu [94].

5.1.3 Composition

The protein quality of soya beans is one of the main reasons for the interest in soya among vegetarians [91]. It has been shown that the quality of soya proteins is very similar to that of cow's milk and egg proteins, which are traditionally used as standard references [95]. A number of scientific studies have been stimulated by the effects of soya protein on health. Compared with other vegetables, soya has a high protein content (36.46g/100g) and a low carbohydrate content (30.16g/100g), making it a unique source of vegetable protein [96]. Soya has the highest content of isoflavones compared with other food sources, and this specificity has beneficial effects on health [97]. Isoflavones, part of a functional class of non-steroidal phytochemicals called phytoestrogens, have a chemical structure and function similar to endogenous oestrogens. Such similarity raises doubts about the use of soya, especially at high doses [98]. Isoflavones are found in several plant sources, such as kidney beans, white beans, red clover and Japanese arrowroot, but only soybeans represent a relevant source [99]. The isoflavone content of soya-based foods varies between brands and preparations. The isoflavones mainly found in soya beans are genistein, daidzein and glycitein. They are widely marketed in the form of food supplements [100, 101].

As well as protein and isoflavones, soya beans contain high levels of PUFAs, B vitamins, fibre, iron (15.7mg/100g), calcium, zinc and other bioactive compounds, making soya a prime candidate for a functional food. Compared with cow's milk, soya beans are considered a good source of calcium (277mg/100g) thanks to their high bioavailability. The soya fibre content (9.3g/100g) is essentially made up of pectic polysaccharides, a type of plant fibre that is easily fermentable by the intestinal microbiota. Soya beans are also a rich source of PUFAs, particularly linolenic acids. In fact, soya is the only source, among the other legumes, to provide considerable quantities of ALA, a ω3 essential fatty acid. The oil contained in soya is made up of 54% LA, 24% oleic acid, 11% palmitic acid, 1 to 9% ALA, with a total saturated fatty acid fraction of 9 to 22%. Soya beans also contain peptides such as lunasin (a 43-amino-acid peptide) and Bowman-Birk (a 71-amino-acid peptide), which are protease inhibitors that have a negative effect on protein digestion and also have a chemopreventive effect in vitro.

Soy proteins and isoflavones have been suggested as the main bioactive components and have received considerable attention. Nevertheless, a wide range of phytochemicals are found in soy, such as phytic acid (1 - 2.2%), sterols (0.23 - 0.46%) and saponins (0.17 - 6.16%) with a wide range of potential health benefits [96].

5.1.4 Therapeutic properties

Of the various soya nutrients, isoflavones and proteins have attracted the most research interest. A health claim, concerning the reduction of coronary heart disease linked to the consumption of soy protein of at least 6.25g per portion with a total of 25g per day, was authorised in 1999 by the FDA. This brought soya to the attention of the food industry. The FDA authorised this claim on the basis of a meta-analysis of the effect of soy protein on serum lipid profile in 38 clinical trials, which showed a relationship between soy consumption and blood levels of total cholesterol, LDL and TG. Subsequently, other countries have published soy claims, such as Canada, Brazil, the UK, Indonesia and the Philippines, mainly for 25g of soy protein as an intervention for cardiovascular protection. Although vegetarians consuming such quantities of soya were very rare, the efficacy of cholesterol lowering in vegetarians has been established. In the same context, an epidemiological study reported that a soy protein intake well below the FDA threshold had a cholesterol-lowering effect. In 2000, a statement for health professionals on the protective activity of soy against coronary heart disease was published by the Nutrition Committee of the American Heart Association. However, in 2012, EFSA declared that there was no cause-effect relationship between isolated soy protein and a reduction in serum LDL concentration. In fact, isoflavone isolate does not appear to be active on blood lipid markers in post-menopausal women. The protein and isoflavone contents of soya are both implicated in the beneficial effects on human health, although interaction with other soya compounds cannot be ruled out [96].

Because of their structural similarity to 17β-estradiol, isoflavones can interact with oestrogen receptors. Through both independent and oestrogen-dependent mechanisms, isoflavones can have beneficial effects on health. Epidemiological studies have found that traditional Asian diets rich in phytoestrogens were associated with a lower risk of coronary heart disease. There is also evidence of a possible benefit in hormone-dependent cancers of the prostate, colon, ovary and breast, menopausal symptoms, obesity, osteoporosis, cognitive dysfunction and reduced overall risk of non-communicable diseases [96, 102, 103]. In addition, soy isoflavones, being a subclass of polyphenols, may also have potential antioxidant properties. These activities are higher in black soya than in their yellow counterparts. Recently, it has been discovered that black soya is richer in gamma-tocopherol, flavonoids and anthocyanins (ATC). As well as being concentrated in the epidermal layer of black soya (more than 2,000 mg/100g) and conferring the dark colour, the latter are responsible for various bioactivities such as antioxidant, anti-apoptotic and anti-inflammatory effects. In subjects whose diet is rich in soya, circulating isoflavone levels can exceed endogenous oestradiol concentrations. Nevertheless, the oestrogenic potency of 17β-oestradiol remains greater than that of isoflavones. In addition, the PUFAs contained in soya could contribute to the protective effects of soya consumption by influencing inflammatory parameters. It has also been suggested that the non-isoflavone components present in soybeans, such as phytic acid and saponins, may have a wide range of bioactivities, including antioxidant, antiviral, anticancer, hepatoprotective and cardiovascular protective effects [96]. In the light of a recent study, it was found that soy-based supplements, by modifying nutritional status and macronutrient and energy intake, can optimise bone health and ensure harmonious physical growth and bone formation [104]. In addition, it has been found that the consumption of soy protein supplements by prepubertal girls and boys can stimulate an increase in height, BMI and weight associated with changes in fat-free mass without affecting sexual maturation or the onset of puberty [105].

5.1.5 Safety profile/Toxicity

In Asian populations, the high consumption of soya-based foods, and therefore of isoflavones, has dispelled critical concerns about the safety of these products. Nevertheless, their use in Western countries and their role in human health remain debatable. Indeed, the consumption of soya can potentially disrupt sex hormones through phytoestrogens and could therefore present a danger, particularly for infants fed a soya-based diet and the putative consequences of a massive introduction of hormones early in life. At present, there are no adverse effects reported from the use of soya-based foods in infants. Nevertheless, the absence of proof is not proof of absence. In addition, soy consumption has been found to be associated with an elevated risk of thyroid disorders, incidence of bladder cancer, dementia, breast cancer and breast cell proliferation. It has also been shown that the use of soya by pregnant women modifies the epigenome in the offspring and may have consequences for the health of stimuli in utero [96, 106].

Although the traditional consumption of soya in Japanese and Chinese diets has a history of safe use, there are some concerns about the use of soya-based foods (such as tofu) on the cognitive system. In one study, a comparison between a diet rich in soya and one low in soya, in the short term, showed no adverse effects on cognitive function and mood in healthy young students. A long-term study showed that daily consumption of 54 mg of genistein in aglycone form by postmenopausal women for 3 years had no effect on thyroid function. In addition, daily consumption of 200 mg of isoflavones for 2 years did not affect TSH. Overall, isoflavones showed a good safety profile for thyroid function. In 2015, an EFSA panel concluded that the intake of 35 to 150 mg per day of isoflavones from supplements or foods had no adverse effects on tissues sensitive to sex hormones such as the uterus and breast or the thyroid gland for up to 2.5 years. In addition, based on clinical and prospective epidemiological data, the use of soy isoflavones by women has been shown to have a good safety profile. A randomised, double-blind, 12-month study showed no worsening of fibroglandular tissue following soy consumption in breast cancer patients previously exposed to antineoplastic treatments or in high-risk women. There are no contraindications to the consumption of isoflavones by women treated with tamoxifen or anastrozole, but an improvement in anticancer treatment has been associated with soy consumption [96]. Although the use of soya-based food supplements as natural alternatives to menopausal hormone therapy has been encouraged, their potential effect on the development of breast cancer is controversial [106]. On the other hand, there is a low prevalence of soy allergy, with rare anaphylactic reactions to soy-containing foods. Generally, soya-based preparations are prescribed as alternatives following adverse reactions to cow's milk. However, clinical manifestations of soy allergy, including enterocolitis, overlap with those of cow's milk allergy. Fermenting soya and soya-based foods reduces allergenicity and immunoreactivity. Compared with cow's milk, soy allergy does not appear to present a danger in human nutrition, even in infants [96].

Overall, an adverse effect of soy intakes on the sex hormone network or the thyroid gland seems unlikely. Traditional soya-based preparations and soya-based foods contain low to moderate levels of bioactive compounds that offer modest health benefits with a very limited risk of potential adverse health effects. To reap the benefits of soya isoflavones, intake should be at least 60-100 mg per day. It is important to label soya-based foods with isoflavone concentrations and inform the consumer in order to take advantage of the health benefits and be vigilant about high intake levels, particularly for long-term consumption [96].

5.2 Chia seeds

5.2.1 Description

Chia, or *Salvia hispanica*, is an annual herbaceous plant that originated in southern Mexico and northern Guatemala. It belongs to the order Lamiales, the mint family *Labiatae*, the subfamily *Nepetoideae* and the genus *Salvia*. The genus *Salvia* includes around 900 species that have been widely distributed in several regions of the world for thousands of years, particularly in southern Africa, Central America, North and South America and south-east Asia [107-113]. *S.hispanica* is commonly known as chia, Spanish sage, Mexican chia and black chia [114]. Today, chia is grown not only in Mexico and Guatemala, but also in Australia, Bolivia, Colombia, Argentina, Peru, America and Europe. Mexico is now recognised as the world's largest producer of chia [112]. *S.hispanica* flowers in summer and produces small (3 to 4 mm), hermaphrodite white and violet flowers. Its leaves are petiolate and inverted serrated, measuring 4 to 8 cm long and 3 to 5 cm wide. It is also sensitive to daylight and can grow up to 1 m high. *S.hispanica* is mainly grown for its seeds, which are generally very small, oval in shape, 2 mm long, 1 to 1.5 mm wide and less than 1 mm thick [108, 109, 112, 115]. Seed colour varies from white to black, grey or mottled black (**Figure 7**).

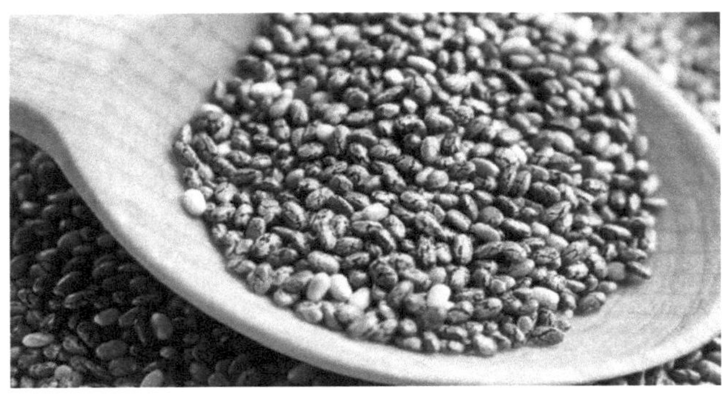

Figure 5 Chia seeds [3]

There is a slight difference between black and white chia seeds that most consider them to be equal. They differ only slightly in morphology: white chia seeds are larger, thicker and wider than black seeds. It's important to note, however, that growing black chia seeds yields around 5% to 8% of white chia seeds at any one time. On the other hand, when only white chia seeds are grown, only white chia seeds are produced **[115]**.

The chia plant is able to grow in a wide range of well-drained clay and sandy soils with reasonable salt and acid tolerance **[116]**. *S.hispanica* can produce 500 to 600 kg of seeds/acre and can even yield 2500 kg/acre under favourable agronomic conditions **[111, 116]**. The word chia comes from '*chian*', a Spanish word meaning oily. According to various sources, chia is an oleaginous seed **[113, 117, 118]**. The chemical composition of chia seeds and their nutritional value can vary depending on various factors such as the year of cultivation, geographical location, climatic conditions, cultivation environment and the extraction method used **[108, 119]**.

5.2.2 History

Chia has been part of the human diet for 5500 years. As recorded in historical archives, *S. hispanica* was used alongside maize, amaranth and beans by the ancient Mesoamerican cultures (Aztecs and Mayans) to prepare traditional foods and medicines. The Aztecs used chia as a source of nourishment and also used it in cosmetics and religious rituals. Moreover, chia was the second most important crop after beans in pre-Columbian societies [111]. The declaration of chia as a functional food by the European Parliament has led to a high level of consumption and an increase in its popularity [120].

Chia seeds are widely used for applications in the food and pharmaceutical industries. They can be found as whole seeds or ground, in the form of flour, oil and gel. In 2000, US guidelines suggested that chia could be used as a primary food in limited quantities, not exceeding 48g/day [109]. Chia seeds can also be added or mixed into biscuits, pasta, cereals, nutritional supplements and cakes. What's more, chia gel and seeds can be used in baked goods as an egg substitute (replacing 25% of eggs) and oil. Being hydrophilic, chia seeds can absorb 12 times their weight in water [109, 119, 120]. Furthermore, by mixing butter with chia oil in a proportion of 6.5% to 25%, the nutritional value of the chia-enriched butter obtained is increased [111]. Today, chia oil is one of the most valuable oils on the market [121]. It has recently been reported that chia mucilage can be used as a foam stabiliser, suspending agent, emulsifier, adhesive or binder due to its water retention capacity and viscosity [111]. Chia seed oil nanoemulsion delivery systems represent a potential as a delivery system for ω-3 fatty acids from chia oil. This represents, in fact, a potential in pharmaceutical, cosmetic and food applications due to the possibility of direct use of emulsions or powder after drying [122].

5.2.3 Composition

Many researchers have analysed the chemical composition of chia seeds. They are a rich source of fat (30 to 33%), carbohydrates (26 to

41%), dietary fibre (18 to 30%), protein (15 to 25%), vitamins, minerals and antioxidants. Chia seeds contain 39% oil (dry seed mass). Several studies have reported that this oil is essentially made up of PUFAs, in particular ALA (ω-3 fatty acids) and LA (ω-6 fatty acids), with levels of up to 68% ALA and 19% LA [109, 113, 117]. As a result, *S.hispanica* is one of the few medicinal plants offered for use in the preparation of omega-3 capsules [123]. Black and white chia seeds have similar chemical compositions: black chia seeds contain 16.9% protein and 32.6% fibre and white chia seeds contain 16.5% protein and 32.4% fibre [115]. The protein content of chia seeds is higher than the protein content of all other cereals (for example, maize (9.4%), rice (6.5%), quinoa (14.1%) and wheat (12.6%)) [111, 124, 125]. The USDA (*United States Department of Agriculture*) has confirmed that chia seeds contain certain exogenous amino acids (arginine, leucine, phenylalanine, vaine and lysine) and certain endogenous amino acids (glutamic and aspartic acids, alanine, serine and glycine) [126]. In addition, chia is highly appreciated by patients suffering from coeliac disease due to the absence of gluten protein [108]. *S.hispanica* is rich in dietary fibre. It contains between 34g and 40g per 100g [108, 111]. Chia seeds are also a good source of minerals such as calcium, phosphorus, potassium, magnesium and vitamins (A, B, K, E, D, mainly vitamins B1, B2 and niacin). The calcium content is higher than that of rice, barley, maize and oats. Compared with other cereals, chia seeds are richer in other minerals such as magnesium, potassium and phosphorus [111, 124]. Concentrating on phenolic content, chia seeds contain 8.8%. Chia seeds also contain high levels of caffeic acid, chlorogenic acid, quercetin, rosmarinic acid, gallic acid, cinnamic acid, myricetin and kaemferol. It also contains isoflavones such as daidzein, glycitein and genistein, in small quantities [121, 127].

5.2.4 Therapeutic properties

The benefits of using chia as a nutritional supplement are enormous [121]. Chia seeds and oil contain a large number of natural antioxidants, such as tocopherols, phytosterols, carotenoids and polyphenolic compounds. Polyphenolic compounds are the most important complexes contributing to the antioxidant activity of chia seeds. They are capable of scavenging free radicals, chelating ions and donating hydrogens [107]. Antioxidant compounds help to reduce the risk of chronic diseases (cancer and heart attack), and provide protection against certain disorders such as diabetes, Alzheimer's and Parkinson's [112]. Several studies have highlighted the antioxidant activity of chia seeds [113, 128-131]. They are therefore considered an excellent example of an antioxidant-rich food. Phytosterols also have antimicrobial and cardio-protective properties [121]. In addition, the ALA contained in chia seeds is capable of blocking the dysfunction of calcium and sodium channels, which can cause hypertension. These PUFAs can also improve heart rate variability and protect against ventricular arrhythmia [132]. In addition, they are hepatoprotective and have anti-inflammatory, anti-diabetic and cholesterol-lowering activities, as well as protecting against cancer, arthritis and autoimmune diseases. LA , in turn, has anti-inflammatory, anti-hypertensive, anti-thrombotic and anti-cancer **activities [108, 109, 111, 112, 133]**. In addition, the chemical compounds found in chia seeds, such as caffeic acid, ferulic acid, chlorogenic acid, rosmarinic acid and flavonoids (quercetin, kaempferol, daidzein, etc.) have different biological activities ranging from antioxidant, anti-ageing and antihypertensive to anticarcinogenic, anti-inflammatory and neuron-protective [109, 121]. In addition, fibre present in large quantities can reduce the risk of coronary heart disease, the risk of T2D and several types of cancer, and its presence in meals helps to reduce subsequent hunger [130].

5.2.5 Safety profile/Toxicity

S.hispanica, being a functional food, is considered safe and without potentially harmful effects [120]. Chia has been shown to have no toxic, anti-nutritional or allergic effects on human health [134, 135]. However, several studies have mentioned that chia seeds are free from mycotoxins and gluten, which are potentially toxic [108, 111]. Dietary supplements with other sources of omega-3 such as flaxseed or marine products generally result in allergy, fishy flavour, diarrhoea and gastrointestinal tract problems. Nevertheless, studies have found that whatever the form of chia, its inclusion did not induce any symptoms of abnormal behaviour, diarrhoea, dermatitis or immuno-nocification effects [136, 137].

Due to the increasing dietary intake of chia and the growing number of authorised uses in recent years, the European Commission recently invited the EFSA Scientific Panel: NDA (*Novel Foods and Foods Allergens*) to give an opinion on the overall safety assessment of chia seeds as a novel food. On the basis of the data provided, previous safety assessments of chia seeds and information extracted from an in-depth literature search carried out by EFSA, the scientific panel came to the conclusion that chia seeds have a good safety profile under the conditions of use evaluated [138]. Despite the existence of several epidemiological and experimental reports promoting the use of chia as an oral supplement, extraction and effective dose protocols need to be standardised to ensure its widespread human consumption and wider therapeutic use, supported by sound scientific data [121].

6 THE LEAVES

6.1 Moringa

6.1.1 Description

Moringa oleifera Lam (*Moringa pterygosperma G.*) is well known as the "pestle tree" because of the appearance of the immature pods, the "horseradish tree" because of the taste of ground root preparations, and the "ben oil tree" because of the oil extracted from its seeds. This plant originally comes from north-west India, its main producer. It is a tree that grows widely in many tropical and sub-tropical countries. It is grown commercially in India, South and Central America, Africa, Mexico, Hawaii and throughout South-East Asia [139, 140].

M.oeifera belongs to the *Moringacae* family, genus *Moringa*. It is the best-known, most widely used and most studied species in its family. There are 14 species in the genus *Moringa*: *M.arborea, M.longituba, M.borziana, M.pygmaea, M.hildebrandtii, M.drouhardii, M.longituba, M.peregrina, M.stenopetala, M.rivae, M.ruspoliana, M.Ovalifolia, M.Concanensis* and *M.oleifera*. The latter is able to survive in hot humid or dry climates and in poor soils [139]. The various parts of *M.oleifera* can be used, including leaves, seeds, immature pods in some regions, bark and roots. However, *M.oeifera* leaves (**Figure 9**) are the most widely used because of their high and important nutritional content [139, 140].

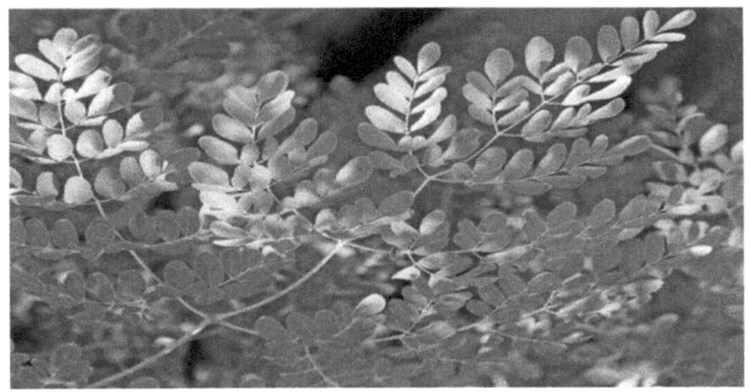

Figure 6: The leaves of *M.oleifera* [141]

6.1.2 History

Moringa has earned the title of 'miracle tree' thanks to its diverse nutritional and therapeutic properties. It is a highly nutritious plant that is considered ideal for treating malnutrition in developing countries. *M.oleifera* has gained commercial attention primarily on the basis of its content of amino acids and flavonoids, which can be of great use in the production of food supplements and cosmetics. In fact, if we compare moringa with other plants and nutritional sources, we find that 100g of dry *M.oleifera* leaves contain 7 times more vitamin C than oranges, 10 times more vitamin A than carrots, 17 times more calcium than milk, 9 times more protein than yoghurt, 15 times more potassium than bananas and 25 times more iron than spinach. It's rare to find so many nutrients in a single plant, and in such large quantities [139]. Because of its richness in nutrients, moringa has attracted a great deal of interest. The content of moringa leaves (FM) varies according to the genetic make-up of the plant, particularly the cultivar and the growing environment [142]. From the leaves to the roots, good quantities of important minerals, proteins, vitamins, β-carotene, amino acids and phenolic compounds can be obtained. Moringa leaves and fruits are commonly used as vegetables in some countries. The FMs can also be dried and used or ground into powder, making them easier to preserve and use. However *M.oleifera* is used or preserved, it does not lose its exceptional nutritional value [139]. As is commonly known, cooking causes most vegetables to lose their nutrients. Nevertheless, it has been found that fresh FM, cooked or preserved dried in powder form for months without refrigeration, still retains its nutritional value. What's more, the iron present in boiled leaves was 3 times more available than that in fresh *M.oleifera* leaves. The same results were found for leaf powder [143].

6.1.3 Composition

The FM contains a greater variety and quantity of proteins than other parts of the plant. On a dry matter basis, one *M.oleifera* leaf contains a crude protein content ranging from 23.0% to 30.3% and a total crude fibre content as low as 5.9%. Compared with soya, which is regarded as a gold standard food, their fibre content is almost equivalent. Another striking feature of FM is its richness in minerals, with a powder content of up to 12%, which is significantly higher than that of soya flour or maize. On a dry matter basis, moringa leaf contains 24700mg/kg of calcium, 4400mg/kg of phosphorus, 318.81 mg/Kg of iron, 190mg/kg of magnesium and 22.05 mg/kg of zinc. Such abundances of minerals in the leaves are relatively high compared with the leaves of other trees. It turns out that FM powder can partially replace milk for children, thanks to its calcium content. Given that iron deficiency is a characteristic generally common to plant-based foods, foods based on FM are the exception. There is 25 times more iron in wolfberries than in spinach. What's more, its absorption rate is higher than that of spinach and other leafy vegetables. FM also contains 7.09% lipids, higher than other woody forage plants. More than half (57%) of the fatty acids in a *M.oleifera* leaf are PUFAs, of which ALA has the highest content. *M.oleifera* also has a high amino acid content. This plant contains 16 to 19 amino acids, including the 10 essential amino acids: threonine, tyrosine, methionine, valine, phenylalanine, isoleucine, leucine, histidine, lysine and tryptophan. In MFs, the complete profile of essential amino acids represents 52.19% of the total amino acids. They are also rich in vitamins, polyphenols (phenolic acids and flavonoids) and carotenoids. In fact, the total phenol and flavonoid content provided by MF is twice that of cabbage, spinach, broccoli, cauliflower and peas [142]. The main flavonoids supplied by *M.oleifera* leaves are myrecytin, quercetin and kaempferol, at concentrations of 5.8, 0.207 and 7.57 mg/g, respectively. Gallic acid is the most abundant phenolic acid present in MF, with a concentration of 1.034mg/g dry weight. In addition, chlorogenic and caffeic acids are present at concentrations ranging from 0.018 to 0.489 mg/g dry weight and 0.409 mg/g dry weight, respectively. Tannins, being water-soluble phenolic compounds, are present in dried moringa leaves at concentrations ranging from 13.2 to 20.6 g tannin/kg [144]. Tannins can be considered anti-nutrients because they interact with trypsin and amylase to form complexes that interfere with digestion. However, drying, fermentation and ensiling reduce tannins by 15 to 30% compared with fresh wake [142]. In addition, an average concentration of 40-139µg/100g of total carotenoids is found in fresh moringa leaves, of which around 47.8% are β-carotenes. These are very important precursors of vitamin A. FMs are also an important source of vitamin E, which has antioxidant properties and boosts cellular immunity, and vitamin C, which is present at a concentration of 200mg/100g [142, 144]. In addition, other compounds have been reported in FM studies, including alkaloids, glucosinolates and isothiocyanates. Saponins are also found in concentrations ranging from 64 to 81 g/kg dry weight of freeze-dried leaves [144]. Saponins are responsible for the bitter taste of FM. Other anti-nutrients, such as phytates and oxalates, can seriously affect the absorption of trace elements in food sources and complicate digestion. However, these two substances are only present in FM at low levels: 22.3 mg/g of dry matter and 27.5 mg/g of dry matter for phytates and oxalates, respectively. This is much lower than in spinach leaves or green pigweed [142].

6.1.4 Therapeutic properties

Given the above nutritional values, *M.oleifera* offers a number of benefits for human health. Due to the high levels of antioxidants present in MFs, they can be used in patients suffering from inflammatory diseases, including cancer, hypertension and CVD. The β-carotene in *M.oleifera* leaves has been shown to act as an antioxidant. According to one study, MF can be an important source of vitamin A for children. It is only when ingested in combination that antioxidants have their maximum effect on the damage caused by free radicals. In fact, a broad combination of antioxidants is found in *M.oleifera* leaves and has been shown to be more effective than a single antioxidant, probably due to synergistic mechanisms. *M.oleifera* leaf extract also provides tannins, saponins, flavonoids, terpenoids and glycosides. These compounds have antioxidant properties and are effective antimicrobial agents. Phenolic compounds act as primary antioxidants. They inactivate lipid free radicals and prevent the decomposition of hydroperoxides into free radicals. In a study of aqueous and ethanolic extracts of freeze-dried *M.oleifera* leaves from different agro-climatic regions, it was found that the different extracts inhibited AL peroxidation by 89.7% to 92%. These extracts also scavenge superoxide radicals. This antioxidant activity varies according to soil properties and ambient temperature [144].

FM extract inhibits the production of cytokines by human macrophages, in particular tumour necrosis factor (TNF-α) and the pro-inflammatory interleukins induced by cigarette smoke and lipopolysaccharide. Similarly, *M.oleifera* concentrate and isothiocyanates have been reported to reduce gene expression and the production of inflammatory markers by macrophages. In cyclophosphamide-induced immunodeficient mice, *M.oleifera* extracts stimulate cellular and humoral immune responses. This activity is ensured by an increase in white blood cells, the percentage of neutrophils and serum immunoglobulins. Quercetin may also be involved in reducing the inflammatory process. In fact, it inhibits the action of transcription factor kappa-beta (NF-kβ) and the events and inflammation that ensue. In addition, fermentation of *M.oleifera* has been shown to improve its anti-inflammatory properties. The presence of quercetin in the methanolic extracts of *M.oleifera* leaves gives this plant a hepatoprotective action. In fact, it has been shown that FM reduces aspartate amino transferase (ASAT), alanine amino transferase (ALAT), alkaline phosphatase and plasma creatinine. They also improve drug-induced liver and kidney damage and reduce lipids and lipid peroxidation levels in rat liver. Similar results were observed in a rat co-treated with FM and NiSO4 to induce nephrotoxicity. In addition, in rats fed a high-fat diet in association with *M.oleifera* leaves, the same reductions in liver enzymes were observed. Furthermore, in a model of hepatic steatosis in guinea pigs, treatment with MF resulted in lower concentrations of hepatic cholesterol and TG in treated animals compared with controls. This lowering of hepatic lipids was accompanied by a reduction in inflammation and in the expression of genes involved in lipid absorption and inflammation. However, no reduction in inflammation was observed in the accumulation of lipids in the adipose tissue of guinea pigs [144].

Almost all parts of the 'miracle tree' have expressed analgesic activity in different animal models. *M.oleifera* leaf extract was found to have unquestionable analgesic activity in central (hot plate method) and peripheral (acetic acid-induced contortion method) models in a dose-dependent manner. FM extracts have been shown to have potent analgesic properties similar to those of indomethacin, as well as anti-migraine properties. Furthermore, in an animal model of LB-induced pyrexia, significant antipyretic activity of FM extract was observed at doses of 100, 200 and 400 mg/kg [145].

Because of the high cost and side-effects of synthetic anti-dementia drugs, there is growing interest in natural products containing flavonoids. These products are considered promising candidates for preventing and/or treating neurodegenerative disorders. It is thought that FM extract has both antioxidant activity and nootropic effects that promote cognitive capacity [146]. As the extract is rich in vitamins C and E, it helps to improve memory in Alzheimer's patients. In addition, the alcoholic extract of FM helps to combat oxidative stress and therefore has a preventive effect on Alzheimer's disease in a rat model of colchicine-induced Alzheimer's disease [145]. *M.oleifera* has been shown to stimulate neuronal growth and survival under difficult treatment conditions. For example, ethanol extract of *M.oleifera* leaves, at a concentration of 30µg/mL, is able to promote neuronal growth and neuronal differentiation of primary embryonic neurons in a concentration-dependent manner. Similarly, *M.oelifera* leaf extract can increase the number and length of dendrites and axon bronchi, the length of axons and can also facilitate synaptogenesis. Previous studies have also shown that *M.oleifera* leaf extract can be an effective remedy as an agent for treating the nervous system and successfully improving memory. It was found that administration of the FM extract at a concentration of 300mg/Kg for 28 consecutive days in rats suffering from AlCl3-induced temporal cortical degeneration reduced the rate of neurotoxicity and the process of neurodegeneration. In the light of a study carried out on standardised mouse models suffering from depression, the antidepressant effect of *M.oleifera* was confirmed. This effect was demonstrated by daily administration of 200 mg/Kg of the alcoholic extract of *M.oleifera* leaves in combination with fluoxetine at a daily dose of 10 mg/Kg for 14 consecutive days. This suggests that a combination of *M.oleifera* and fluoxetine or other selective serotonin reuptake inhibitors (SSRIs) may have promising potential **[146]**.

Following supplementation with aqueous extract of FM at a dose of 100 mg/Kg, an improvement in insulin sensitivity, an increase in total antioxidant capacity and better immune tolerance were observed. This is consistent with another report which indicates that *M.oleifera* is capable of improving glucose intolerance. It may also reduce the complications associated with diabetes. In fact, using control and diabetic rats whose diabetes was induced by streptozotocin, it was found that administration of FM extract (250 mg/Kg) for 6 weeks played a key role in reducing diabetic complications. This is by protecting the renal lesions and inflammation induced by diabetes **[146]**. Several compounds provided by *M.oleifera* leaves may be involved in glucose homeostasis. For example, isothiocyanates have been reported to reduce insulin resistance and hepatic gluconeogenesis. Phenolic acids and flavonoids also influence β-cell mass and function and increase insulin sensitivity in peripheral tissues. In addition, phenolic compounds, flavonoids and tannins inhibit intestinal sucrase and pancreatic α-amylase activities **[144]**. In addition, several compounds in FMs are used in blood pressure stabilisation, including nitrile, mustard oil glycosides and thiocyanate glycosides. The 4 pure compounds isolated from the ethanolic extract of *M.oleifera* leaves, niazinin A, niazinin B, niazimicin and niazinin A+B, have been found to have a hypotensive effect in rats, probably mediated by a calcium antagonist effect. A recent study reported that *M.oleifera* reduced vascular oxidation in spontaneously hypertensive rats **[144]**.

They contain phenolic compounds and flavonoids that play an important role in lipid regulation by inhibiting the activity of pancreatic cholesterol esterase. In this way, they reduce and delay cholesterol absorption and form complexes with bile acids for excretion. In rats fed a high-fat diet, it was thought that the β-sitosterol contained in FMs was responsible for the drop in plasma cholesterol in the animals tested. By binding to cholesterol and bile acids, the saponins found in *M.oleifera* leaves in turn prevent the absorption of cholesterol and increase faecal excretion of bile acids and reduce their enterohepatic circulation. To compensate for the increased elimination of bile acids, the body carries out improved synthesis of bile acids from cholesterol in the liver, which lowers plasma cholesterol **[144]**. On the other hand, several studies have reported that extracts of *M.oleifera* leaves have properties that effectively inhibit the growth of breast, pancreatic and colorectal cancer cells. Indeed, *M.oleifera* has attracted a great deal of interest for its chemoprotective properties. FMs have the ability to protect organisms and cells against oxidative DNA damage associated with cancer and degenerative diseases. FM extract has been shown to inhibit the viability of acute myeloid leukaemia, acute lymphoblastic leukaemia and hepatocellular carcinoma cells. This anti-cancer activity is linked to several bioactive compounds in FM, including isothiocyanate, niazimicin and β-sitosterol. FM extract has been shown to limit the spread of pancreatic cancer cells by inhibiting transcription in cancer cells, while increasing the efficacy of chemotherapy in these cells. Similar antiproliferative effects have also been demonstrated in breast cancer cells **[144]**.

6.1.5 Safety profile/Toxicity

No adverse effects have been reported in human studies. Various preparations of M.oleifera have been used traditionally and are still used throughout the world as foods and medicines without any adverse effects being reported. The potential toxicity of *M.oleifera* leaves has been assessed in several animal trials [140].

A study in albino Wistar mice reported that an aqueous extract of FM caused no mortality at oral doses of up to 6400 mg/Kg. In rats, higher doses (3200 and 6400 mg/Kg) triggered dullness and reduced locomotion. No significant differences were observed in the quality of the rats' sperm or in their histological, biochemical or haematological parameters. The LD50 limit dose was determined to be 1585/mg/Kg. In another study, micro-nucleated polychromatic erythrocytes were found in the bone marrow of the femur of Sprague-Dawley rats following administration of high doses of FM (3000 mg/Kg). This study reported that, because of the high concentrations of nitrogen compounds in *M. oleifera*, doses of over 3000mg/Kg can cause acute toxicity and an increase in urea levels in rats [147]. In a series of experiments, the cytotoxicity of an aqueous extract of FM was assessed by exposing human peripheral blood mononuclear cells in vitro to graded doses of the extract. Cytotoxicity was observed at 20mg/Kg, a concentration that cannot be achieved per os. Several animal toxicity studies report that *M.oleifera* dried leaf extract can be safe for consumption, although at high doses and prolonged intakes, it can be toxic through accumulation of certain elements. It is therefore recommended not to exceed a maximum dose of 70g/day [139].

6.2 Green tea

6.2.1 Description
These days, tea is ranked as the second most widely consumed beverage in the world, just after water. The tea plant is called *Camillia sinensis* and belongs to *the Theaceae* family. Black tea, oolong tea and green tea (**Figure 9**) are the three main forms of tea and are produced from the leaves of *C.sinensis*. It is an evergreen shrub or tree that is

generally pruned to 2-5 feet for cultivation, but can reach a height of 30 feet. Its leaves are dark green, oval with serrated edges. Its flowers are white, fragrant and appear singly or in clusters. Since the 3 types of tea mentioned above come from the same *C.sinensis* plant, the difference lies in the way the leaves are processed. The 3 types of tea are classified according to the level of antioxidants and the degree of fermentation. Unlike black and oolong, green tea is produced without oxidising the young tea leaves. Green tea is produced by steaming fresh leaves at high temperatures, which inactivates the oxidising enzymes. This keeps the polyphenol content intact and protects most of the vitamins present. As a result, green tea is richer in antioxidants than other teas **[148, 149]**.

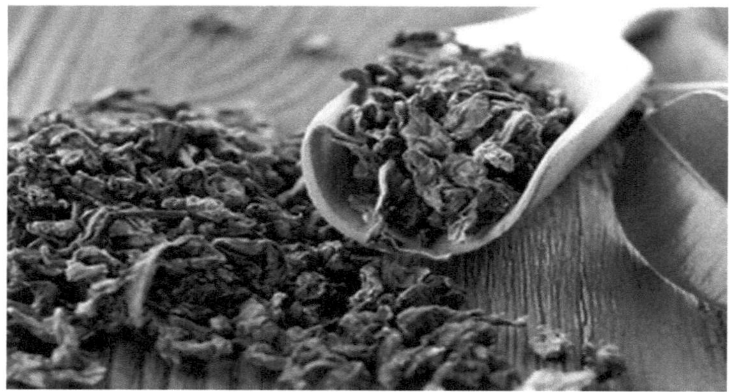

Figure 7 Green tea leaves [150]

6.2.2 History

Based on the available literature, tea was first consumed as a beverage or medicine by the Chinese population around 2737 BC **[149]**. The first green tea was exported from India to Japan in the 17th century **[151]**. Today, tea is consumed in almost every country in the world. The main tea producers are China, India and Kenya. Tea is grown on all six continents, and around 3 billion kilos of tea are produced and consumed worldwide each year **[149]**. The biggest consumers of tea are the inhabitants of Europe, mainly Great Britain, who consume around

540ml of tea a day. However, the average person in the world consumes around 120ml/day **[149]**. Today, green tea is also used in the preparation of various foods, pharmaceutical preparations and cosmetics **[151]**.

6.2.3 Composition

Green tea contains mainly polyphenols (90%), amino acids (7%), proanthocyanidins and caffeine (3%). Catechins and flavonols (myricetin, caempherol, quercetin, chlorogenic acid, coumarylquinic acid and theogallin) are the main polyphenols found in green tea **[150]**. The catechin group (flavan-3-ol) is part of the flavonoid group. Flavonoids are one of the most common and varied groups of polyphenols(309). The main catechins present are catechin (C), epicatechin (EC), gallocatechin (GC), epigallocatechin (EGC), epicatechin gallate (GEC), epigallocatechin gallate (GEGC) and gallocatechin gallate (GCG). Of the catechins mentioned, 80% of all green tea catechins are made up of GEGC, GEC and EGC **[152]**.

The percentage content of tea is variable and depends on various environmental factors, including growing conditions, soil, climatic conditions and other external factors such as light, geography, microbes and temperature **[152]**. In addition, the time of harvest and the age of the leaves are factors that influence tea quality. During subsequent harvests, the quantity of theanine, theobromine, caffeine, catechin and GCG decreases. However, under the same conditions, there is an increase in EC, GEGC and EGC. Similarly, young leaves (up to the 7th leaf) were found to contain higher levels of caffeine, GEGC, GEC and other catechins than older leaves. This is probably due to the wilting process. The most abundant catechin in *C.sinensis* is GEGC, which accounts for 50-80% of total catechins. This substance is thought to be the main contributor to the various health benefits of green tea. Based on EFSA data, 100ml of green tea corresponds to 126mg of catechins. According to the FDA, there are 71 mg of GEGC in 100 mL of green tea. In addition, there are chlorogenic acid and coumarylquinic acid, as well as theogaline (3-galloylquinic acid) and theanine (5-N-ethylglutamine). These 4 substances are found exclusively in tea. There are also traces of other common methylxanthines, theobromine and theophylline. Tea is also capable of accumulating aluminium and manganese. Depending on the fermentation process and the age and size of the tea leaves, several minerals such as fluoride, zinc, chromium, selenium, calcium and magnesium are present in tea leaves in varying concentrations [149].

6.2.4 Therapeutic properties

In ancient Asian folk medicine, tea was considered an effective medicine for the treatment of various ailments. Green tea has attracted a great deal of attention, mainly because of its exceptional richness in antioxidants, making it a key regulator of free radicals. In fact, it is considered a functional food because it can confer numerous physiological benefits in addition to its nutritional content [149]. The antioxidant potential of green tea is influenced by the technological process of treatment. In fact, green tea is much richer in catechins than black tea, since fermentation of the latter results in oxidation of the catechins to theaflavins. It's important to note, however, that the higher the catechin content of the tea, the higher the antioxidant activity. In addition, increasing the temperature increases the antioxidant activity of the green tea infusion [152]. By protecting against oxidants and free radicals, green tea also strengthens the immune system. It also inhibits lipid peroxidation. This effect was also observed in the kidney after oral administration of the main polyphenol in green tea, GEGC. In addition, green tea, its extract and its constituents have been shown to prevent oxidative stress and neurological problems. Green tea also has a chemopreventive effect on cigarette smokers. In addition to its antioxidant activity, the constituents of green tea have antimutagenic and anticarcinogenic effects and may protect humans against the risk of cancer caused by environmental agents. Indeed, green tea consumption has been found to protect against many types of cancer, including those of the lung, colon, oesophagus, mouth, stomach, small intestine, kidney, pancreas and mammary glands [151]. There is abundant in vivo evidence to confirm that drinking green tea or taking it as a dietary supplement has anti-cancer properties. However, it must be clearly emphasised that green tea and catechins cannot replace standard chemotherapy [152]. To demonstrate the effects of green tea against breast cancer, a case-control study was carried out in south-east China between 2004 and 2005. There were 1009 patients aged between 20 and 87 with histologically confirmed breast cancer and 1009 healthy control women of the same age randomly recruited from breast disease clinics. Information was collected on the duration, frequency, quantity, preparation and type of tea consumption as well as diet and lifestyle. It was found that green tea drinkers tended to live in urban areas, were better educated and consumed more coffee, alcohol, soya, vegetables and fruit. After adjusting for established and potential confounding factors, green tea consumption was found to be associated with a reduced risk of breast cancer. Similar dose-response relationships were observed for duration of tea consumption, number of cups consumed and new batches prepared per day. In addition, studies of animal models have shown that the catechins in green tea offer some protection against degenerative diseases. In some studies, green tea was found to have antiproliferative activity on hepatoma and hypolipidaemic activity in rats treated for hepatoma, as well as preventing hepatotoxicity. In addition to their antimutagenic activity, green tea catechins are also considered to be immune modulators of immunodysfunction caused by transplanted tumours or by carcinogenic treatment. In chronic liver disease, the proliferation of hepatic fibrosis is closely linked to the proliferation of hepatic star cells. GEGC has a potential inhibitory effect on these cells. Recent studies have suggested that green tea polyphenols may protect against Parkinson's, Alzheimer's and other neurodegenerative diseases. In addition, green tea polyphenols have been shown to have neuroprotective activity in cell cultures and animal models, such as preventing neurotoxin-induced cell damage **[151]**.

In the light of several epidemiological studies and clinical trials, green tea has been shown to reduce the risk of many chronic diseases. These effects are attributed to the presence of polyphenols, which are powerful antioxidants. In particular, green tea lowers blood pressure and reduces the risk of stroke and coronary heart disease. Some animal studies have suggested that green tea may protect against the development of coronary heart disease by reducing blood sugar levels and body weight. However, these data are based on middle-aged animal populations, and not on elderly populations whose nutritional status is more likely to be influenced by biological factors **[151]**.

The effectiveness of green tea in treating typhoid and all types of diarrhoea has been well known in Asia since ancient times. The catechins in green tea effectively inhibit *Helicobacter pylori* infections. Green tea has also been shown to be effective against the *herpes simplex* virus and the influenza virus, particularly in the early stages. Green tea catechins also inhibit adenovirus infection in vitro. One study highlighted the antifungal effect of green tea catechins against *Candida albicans*. This study also suggested combining catechins with lower doses of antimycotics to avoid the side effects of antimycotics **[151]**.

Green tea consumption is associated with an increase in bone mineral density. In fact, it has been identified as an independent protective factor against the risk of hip fractures. Several studies have demonstrated the positive effects of green tea extracts and its polyphenols on the proliferation and activity of bone cells. In an experimental system, green tea was found to act by preserving the antioxidant defence system of the crystalline lens [151]. In addition, supplementation with decaffeinated green tea extract has been shown to have beneficial effects on haemodialysis-induced reactive oxygen species, risk factors for atherosclerotic disease and pro-inflammatory cytokines. The pharmacokinetics of an oral dose of catechins were compared between healthy subjects and haemodialysis patients. The antioxidant effects of three different doses (0, 455 and 910 mg) of oral catechins were compared with those of oral vitamin C (500 mg) during a haemodialysis session. Patients supplemented with catechins showed a reduction in plasma hypochlorous acid activity promoted by haemodialysis, more effectively than placebo or vitamin C. Between treatments with 455 and 910 mg of catechins, there was no significant difference in the reduction of plasma hypochlorous acid activity. Catechins also significantly reduced the expression of pro-inflammatory cytokines enhanced by haemodialysis [151]. Studies of the thermogenic properties of green tea have shown that there is a synergistic interaction between caffeine and catechins, which appear to prolong the sympathetic stimulation of thermogenesis. Based on a human study of green tea extract containing 90mg of GEGC administered 3 times a day, it was concluded that men taking the extract burned 266 more calories per day than those taking the placebo. It has also been suggested that the thermogenic effects of green tea may play a role in controlling obesity. Similarly, tea polyphenols have been shown to clearly inhibit digestive lipases in vitro, leading to a reduction in TG lipolysis and therefore possibly reduced fat digestion in humans [148].

6.2.5 Safety profile/Toxicity

Generally speaking, green tea is considered to be a safe, non-toxic beverage, and there are generally no side effects. Depending on the clinical situation and the desired therapeutic effect, the dosage of green tea varies. It is generally recommended to consume 3 to 10 cups of tea a day, although the cancer-preventing effects are generally associated with the higher doses [148].

Green tea offers a number of undeniable benefits for human health, but the effects of green tea and its constituents are beneficial up to a certain dose. With higher doses, unknown undesirable effects may be caused. What's more, the catechins in green tea produce effects that may not manifest themselves in the same way in all individuals. GEGC extracted from green tea is cytotoxic, so consuming high doses of green tea can induce acute cytotoxicity in liver cells, an essential metabolic organ in the body. Another study revealed that higher consumption of green tea may cause oxidative damage to DNA in the pancreas and hamster liver. One study clarified that GEGC acts as a pro-oxidant, rather than an antioxidant, in pancreatic β cells in vivo. Therefore, over-consumption of green tea may be detrimental to diabetic animals in controlling hyperglycaemia. When green tea extract was tested at a high dose (5% of the diet for 13 weeks), thyroid hypertrophy (goitre) was observed in normal rats. With this high-dose treatment, changes in thyroid hormones were observed. However, it is unlikely to cause such adverse effects in humans, even when drinking very large quantities of green tea [151].

There are three main factors associated with the harmful effects of over-consumption of green tea: its caffeine content, the presence of aluminium and the effects of tea polyphenols on iron availability. Patients with heart problems or major cardiovascular problems should not drink green tea **[151]**. During pregnancy or when breast-feeding, women should not drink more than one or two cups a day, as caffeine can increase the heart rate and cause certain disorders such as insomnia, irritability, nervousness and sleep disorders in infants **[148, 151]**. Because of the diuretic effects of caffeine, it is important to control the concomitant consumption of green tea and certain medications. Several studies have revealed the capacity of tea plants to accumulate high levels of aluminium. This is of great importance for patients with renal failure, as aluminium, when accumulated by the body, can lead to neurological diseases. It is therefore necessary to control the consumption of foods containing high levels of this metal. Similarly, the affinity of green tea catechins for iron may significantly reduce the bioavailability of iron from food **[151]**.

7 MACA ROOTS

7.1 Description

Lepidium meyenii Walpers (maca) is a Peruvian plant that grows to heights of over 4,000 metres and has great bioprospecting potential. Maca belongs to the brassica (mustard) family and to the genus *Lepidium*, which is one of the largest genera in the *Brassicaceae* family. Among the most relevant plants associated with *L.meyenii* are rapeseed, mustard, turnip, black mustard, cabbage and watercress. The species from North America and Europe has been extensively studied, while *L.meyenii* from the Andean region has recently been extensively studied for its health benefits. Maca is a very hardy plant that grows on high peaks, in a habitat of intense cold, extremely intense sun and strong winds [153].

The maca plant consists of an aerial part and an underground part. The above-ground part is small and flat in appearance. This is probably the result of a process of adaptation to avoid the impact of the strong winds of the high mountains. The underground part is the hypocotyl-root axis. The main part of the plant, which is also the edible part, is a radish-shaped tuber that forms the hypocotyl and root of the plant. This hypocotyl-root axis is 10 to 14 cm long and 3 to 5 cm wide. It is, in fact, the storage organ that retains a high water content in the form of stock. After natural drying, the hypocotyls are considerably reduced in size to around 2 to 8 cm in diameter (**Figure 10**). Similarly, the average weight of dried hypocotyls varies considerably. For example, in the central Peruvian Andes, we found a weight range of between 7.64 and 23.88 g. There is a variable range of maca types that can be characterised on the basis of the colour of their hypocotyls. 13 colours of maca have been described, ranging from white to black in Carhuamayo, Junin, in the Peruvian highlands. In fact, it has recently been shown that different types of maca (depending on colour) have different biological properties [153].

As demand for the maca plant has grown, traditional cultivation methods have been replaced by mass production practices involving the use of fertilisers and pesticides. Indeed, maca is now grown in regions other than the Andes, such as Yunnan province in China. Such changes could potentially affect the phytochemistry and composition of the plant, and therefore the quality, safety and efficacy of maca products [154].

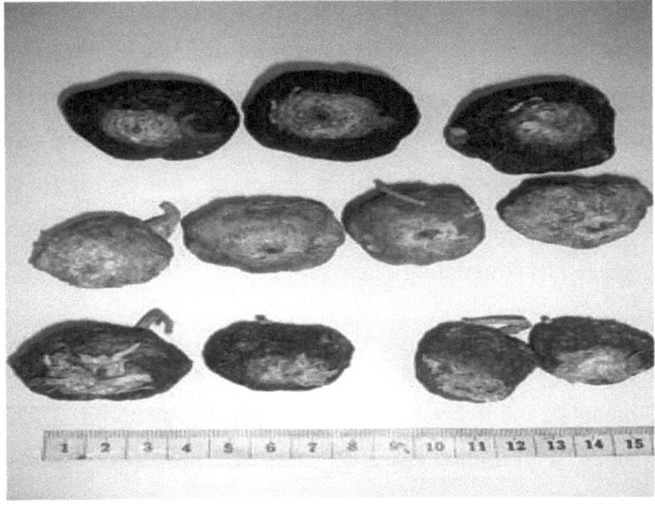

Figure 8: Dried maca [153]

7.2 History

For centuries, maca has been used in the Andes for nutrition and for its benefits for humans and animals. Indeed, *L.meyenii* has traditionally been used as a tonic, improving fertility in humans and cattle, and for the treatment of a variety of illnesses such as rheumatism, respiratory disorders and anaemia, among others. Maca root is cooked, baked, fermented as a drink and made into porridge [154]. Maca was cultivated in the central Peruvian Andes, in the ancient Chinchaycocha (Bombon Plateau) now known as Carhuamayo, Junin and Ondores in the Junin Plateau near Cerro de Pasco. The domestication of maca probably took place between 1300 and 2000 years ago, in San Blas, Junin (today: Ondores). In 1553, a description of maca as a root was published for the first time, without identifying its botanical or popular name. In this publication, Cieza de Leon, a chronicler of the Spanish conquest of Peru, mentioned that a certain root was used by the natives in the Peruvian highlands, particularly in the province of Bombon (Chinchaycocha or as it is known today, Junin) for maintenance. The roots he mentioned were indeed those of maca. The first description of the name maca and its properties was in 1653 by Father Cobo. He stated that this species grows in the harshest and coldest regions of the province of Chinchaycocha, where no other plant could be cultivated for human subsistence. Cobo did, however, mention its use for fertility. Indeed, in the $18^{\text{ème}}$ century, Ruiz spoke of maca's fertility-enhancing activities and its stimulating effect [153].

7.2.1 Composition

Maca contains primary metabolites, corresponding to the nutritional components of the hypocolytes, and secondary metabolites, which are compounds with biological and medicinal properties. In terms of primary metabolites, dried maca hypocotyls contain around 13-16% protein, and are extremely rich in essential amino acids. Fresh hypocotyls are also extremely rich in water (80%) and contain high levels of iron and calcium. The chemical composition of dried maca described in more detail shows: 10.2% protein, 59% carbohydrates, 2.2% lipids and 8.5% fibre. There are also fatty acids, the most abundant of which are AL, palmitic and oleic. The saturated fatty acid content is 40.1%, while the unsaturated fatty acid content is 52.7%. The amino acids contained in maca (mg/g protein) include: leucine (91mg), arginine (99.4mg), phenylalanine (55.3 mg), lysine (54.3 mg), glycine (68.3 mg), alanine (63.1 mg), valine (79.3 mg), isoleucine (47.4 mg), glutamic acid (156.5 mg), serine (50.4 mg) and aspartic acid (47.4 mg). Other amino acids are also present but in lower concentrations, such as histidine (21.9 mg), threonine (33.1 mg), tyrosine (30.6 mg), methionine (28 mg), hydroxyproline (26 mg), proline (0.5 mg) and sarcosine (0.7 mg). Maca also contains minerals, including iron (16.6 mg/100g dry matter), calcium (150 mg/100g dry matter), copper (5.9 mg/100g dry matter), zinc (3.8 mg/100g dry matter) and potassium (2050 mg/100g dry matter) [153].

Maca also contains a variety of secondary metabolites. The secondary metabolites macaridin, macaenes, macamides and alkaloids are found exclusively in maca. Macaenes are unsaturated fatty acids. There are also other compounds containing sterols, such as beta-sitosterol, campesterol and stigmasterol. Various glucosinolates have been described in maca, such as the aromatic glucosinolate glucotropeoline. Benzyl glucosinolate has been suggested as a marker of maca's biological activity. However, this suggestion has been dismissed because glucosinolates can be readily metabolised to isothiocyanates and other smaller metabolites. Benzyl glucosinolate is also found in another Peruvian plant called mashua (*Tropaeolum tuberosum*). It has been noted that maca batches from different producers vary considerably in terms of macaene, macamides, sterols and glucosinolates. It was in 2005 that it was first stated in a publication that different types of maca colour have different properties. More recently, it has been found that maca colours are associated with variations in the concentrations of distinct bioactive metabolites. These compounds, acting individually or synergistically, are capable of acting to promote the reported biological properties of maca. The different colours of maca are therefore linked to differences in the proportion of secondary metabolites, which explains the different biological effects described for maca. Furthermore, it seems that the boiling process increases the active metabolites. The availability of several of the plant's secondary metabolites increases with temperature [153].

7.3 Therapeutic properties

Nowadays maca is widely used as a food supplement because of its various medicinal properties [153]. Indeed, following the introduction of maca to the world market over the last twenty years, there has been a remarkably large increase in demand for this plant over this period, with it being promoted on the internet under the name "Peruvian ginseng" for improving libido and fertility. There was also talk of its potential in treating menopausal symptoms, erectile dysfunction and benign prostatic hyperplasia. Meanwhile, research into the medicinal properties of maca has followed the peak in popularity and has focused mainly on the plant's fertility-enhancing aphrodisiac properties [154].

Maca has been reported to improve sexual behaviour in laboratory animals, although conflicting results have been observed. In a randomised study, it was not possible to demonstrate the effect of maca on penile erection in apparently healthy adult men after 12 weeks of treatment with gelatinised maca, compared with results using a placebo [153]. In addition, a systematic review of the effect of maca on male sexual function was carried out, including four randomised clinical trials (RCTs). Based on two RCTs, it was suggested that maca has a significant positive effect on sexual dysfunction or sexual desire in healthy postmenopausal women or healthy adult men, respectively. However, no effect was observed in the other RCT in healthy cyclists. Nevertheless, analysis of the results of this study showed that maca extract had a significant boosting effect on the self-assessed sexual desire score compared with the baseline test and the placebo trial after supplementation. This effect was observed after 14 days of treatment in this study, which is significantly shorter than that shown with gelatinised maca, where the effects were observed after 8 weeks of treatment. Another RCT evaluating the effects of maca in patients with mild erectile dysfunction used the International Index of Erectile Function-5 (IIFE-5) and showed significantly significant effects on subjective perception of general and sexual well-being. In a placebo-free study, maca was administered in two doses (1.5 g/day and 3 g/day) to patients with SSRI-induced sexual dysfunction. The *Arizona* Sexual *Experiences* Scale (ASEX) and the *Massachusetts General Hospital* Sexual Function Questionnaire (MGH-SFQ) were used to measure sexual dysfunction. Significant improvements in the ASEX and MGH-SFQ scores were observed in subjects taking 3 g/day of maca, but not in subjects taking 1.5 g/day of maca. Similarly, there was a significant improvement in libido based on ASEX number 1. Maca was well tolerated. Given that several pieces of evidence suggest an effect of maca on sexual desire and mild erectile dysfunction, there is also data revealing that maca extract seems to have a better effect than gelatinised maca and maca flour. It is likely that this difference is due to the fact that the extract concentrates the secondary metabolites. In conclusion, there is evidence that maca is capable of improving sexual desire but no conclusive effect on erectile function [153].

In addition to the clinical trials that have shown maca to be effective in treating sexual dysfunction, it has also been implicated in increasing spermatogenesis and sperm mobility [155]. In one study, maca was administered for 4 months to 9 apparently healthy men. An increase in seminal volume, sperm count and sperm motility was observed. However, there was no impact on serum hormone levels, including LH, FSH, prolactin, oestradiol and testosterone, in any of the men tested. Scientific evidence also suggests that maca can be an energiser. Maca has been shown to reduce depression and anxiety scores. A self-perception survey showed that maca may act as an energiser compared with placebo in apparently healthy men [153].

A randomised trial was conducted in patients with metabolic syndrome to assess the effect of maca and yacon in combination with silymarin. The study lasted 90 days and was placebo-controlled. Plasma and lipoprotein lipids, blood glucose and safety parameters were assessed in patients with metabolic syndrome. No adverse effects were found in volunteers using silymarin (0.8 g/day), silymarin + yacon (0.8 + 2.4 g/day) and silymarin + maca (0.6 + 0.2 g/day). However, a moderate ASAT level and an increase in diastolic blood pressure were observed in volunteers using maca (0.6 g/day) [153]. One study found that populations consuming maca had reduced serum levels of interleukin-6, which was associated with lower systolic blood pressure, a higher health score and a lower chronic mountain sickness score [155]. In a randomised clinical trial in healthy men, gelatinised maca was shown to reduce systolic and diastolic blood pressure after 12 weeks of treatment. What's more, maca has been shown to significantly inhibit angiotensin I-converting enzyme linked to hypertension in vitro. Indeed, in populations traditionally consuming maca, systolic blood pressure was found to be lower than in those not consuming maca. Similarly, ASAT levels were similar in maca consumers and non-consumers. Because it is rich in potassium, an important nutrient for reducing the risk of hypertension, maca appears to be of great benefit to patients suffering from hypertension. Other secondary metabolites of maca may also be active in reducing blood pressure [153].

Although there is no traditional description of maca's effect on learning and memory, the indigenous people of Peru's central Andes attribute improved school performance to the consumption of maca by children.

In fact, experimental studies have shown that black maca has beneficial effects on learning and memory in experimental animal models. We studied 3 varieties of maca (yellow, red and black), and found that only black maca had significant biological effects on memory. We studied hydroalcoholic extracts or a boiled extract of maca. Both were similarly effective in improving memory and learning. Black maca (0.5 and 2 g/KG) reduced levels of cerebral malondialdehyde, a marker of oxidative stress, and acetylchilinesterase levels in ovariectomised mice. But there was no difference in monoamine oxidase levels. Black maca appears to improve experimental memory disorders induced by ovariectomy, orchiectomy, scopolamine and alcohol [153].

In addition, a randomised double-blind study was carried out on 95 patients suffering from osteoarthritis. A combination of 300 mg *Uncaria guianensis* (cat's claw) and 1500 mg maca was administered twice a day for 8 weeks. The results were compared with those of treatment with glucosamine sulphate. A considerable improvement in patients' pain, stiffness and function was noted in both types of treatment. However, as the study did not include a placebo control group, the effects of glucosamine remain uncertain [153].

7.4 Safety profile/Toxicity

For centuries, the Peruvian population of the central Andes have used hypocotyls after they have been naturally dried and in quantities >20g/day. No adverse effects have been reported following consumption of *L.meyenii* in food [153]. In the Peruvian population of Carhuamayo, maca users aged between 35 and 74 showed no deterioration in their health with age [155]. Nevertheless, it is recommended by the indigenous people of the Peruvian highlands that maca be boiled before consumption, as fresh maca can have harmful effects on health. The effects of fresh maca on health have not yet been scientifically evaluated [153].

On the basis of the above review data on in vivo and in vitro studies with maca, it appears that the use of maca is safe. There is further evidence that aqueous and methanolic extracts of maca do not exhibit hepatotoxicity in vitro. In addition, administration of freeze-dried aqueous extract of maca (1g/kg body weight) to mice revealed no toxic effect on the normal development of pre-implantation mouse embryos. In rats, different types of maca (black, red and yellow) were found to have no acute toxicity at a dose $\leq$ 17 g dried hypocotyl / Kg body weight. Chronic treatment of rats for 84 days with 1 g/Kg body weight showed no side effects and a histological picture of the liver similar to that of control rats. On the basis of animal studies, a dose of 1 to 2 g/Kg body weight is considered safe. In fact, consumption $\leq$ 1 g/Kg per day is considered safe for humans. Nevertheless, as indicated above in a study of patients with metabolic syndrome, maca consumption at a dose of 0.6 g/day for 90 days resulted in an increase in AST and diastolic blood pressure. These effects have not been confirmed in other studies. Data from a population of 600 subjects in the central Peruvian Andes showed that maca consumption was safe and beneficial to health [153].

To date, further scientific research into maca is required as maca's health claims cannot be sufficiently substantiated from a scientific point of view. To meet the demands of a growing market for herbal remedies, it seems that local indigenous knowledge about the health benefits of maca has been taken out of context. This has serious consequences for local producers in Peru. The lack of protocols to regulate and control the production and marketing of maca during this rapid expansion poses a threat to both consumer safety and the sustainability of the supply [154].

8 RED FRUIT

8.1 Description

The term "red fruit" or "berries" is used to describe the small, sweet or bitter, juicy and intensely coloured fruits (usually red, purple or blue) that grow on wild bushes. If there are no objectionable seeds, they can be eaten whole. The best-known and most widely studied red fruits include strawberries (*Fragaria x ananassa*), raspberries (*Rubus idaeus*), bilberries (*Vaccinium corymbosum*), blackberries (*Rubus fruticosus*) and cranberries *(Vaccinium macrocarpon)*. There are also other less common fruits that are considered to be red fruits, such as cherries, blackberries, blackcurrants and elderberries **[156]**. Red fruits (**Figure 11**) are commonly characterised by the presence of bioactive chemical compounds (TCAs) that produce natural pigments responsible for the colours blue, violet, red, black and orange.

In recent years, red berries have become increasingly important to consumers and industry alike. A number of studies have focused on analysing the composition and pharmacological properties of berries, as well as optimal extraction methods. The aim is to obtain the maximum extraction yield of the compounds of interest that are likely to have the greatest health benefits. Although the conventional solvent extraction method is the most widely used technique for extracting bioactives from soft fruits, there are new non-conventional methods recommended as environmentally friendly alternatives to the old method, such as ultrasound, microwave and pressure-assisted extraction **[156]**.

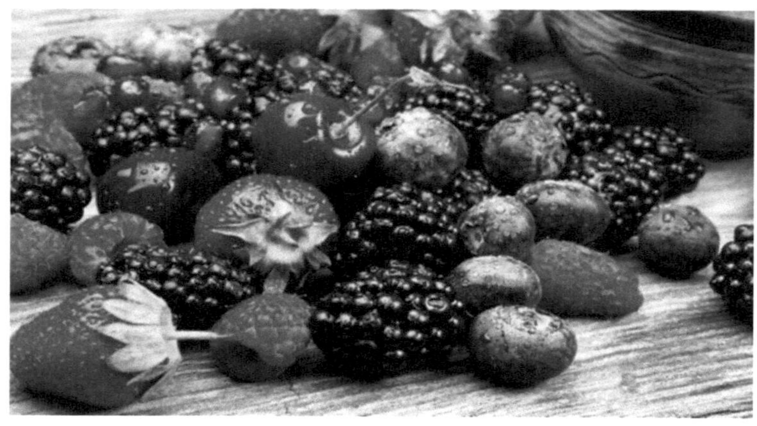

Figure 9: Red fruit [157]

8.2 History

In recent years, the consumption of red fruit has increased remarkably worldwide. Not only are they now eaten fresh, but they are also used in cosmetics and food supplements. A concentrate rich in active molecules, particularly antioxidants, is extracted from edible berries to produce nutraceuticals, creams and functional foods [156].

8.2.1 Composition

There are over 5,000 individual phytochemical compounds in fruit and vegetables. There are 5 main categories: phenolics, carotenoids, alkaloids, nitrogen compounds and organosulphur compounds. Phenolics or polyphenols, being the largest group of phytochemical compounds, contain 5 sub-categories: phenolic acids, stilbenes, coumarins, tannins and flavonoids. One of the characteristics of berries is their richness in antioxidant molecules (polyphenols), which protect the fruit against oxidation caused by environmental factors such as light, air, oxygen and microbiological attack. Bilberries and cranberries are the richest berries in antioxidants. Phenolic acids are divided into two categories: hydroxybenzoic acid derivatives and hydroxycinnamic acid derivatives. The first group includes molecules such as hydroxybenzoic, gallic, vanillic and ellagic acid. The second group includes p-coumaric acid, caffeic acid, ferric acid, chlorogenic acid and hydroxycinnamic acid. These compounds are widely found in berries and each type of berry is defined by a characteristic profile of phenolic molecules [156]. TCAs are a major class of flavonoids. They are a type of water-soluble polyphenol that produce natural pigments characteristic of red berries and have several important therapeutic properties [158]. These natural colourants have little or no toxicity and are commonly used in the food industry. TCA-based colourings are used in drinks, yoghurts and certain fruit juices. They are, in fact, a better alternative to synthetic colourings because they can be consumed safely even in higher doses than synthetic colourings, which can be toxic. What's more, as natural colourings, TCAs offer value-added properties. Recently, acylated TCAs have been recommended for use as food colours because they are more stable than non-acylated TCAs [159]. Anthocyanidins are based on either the flavylium ion or 2-phenylchromenylium. In nature, there are around 17 anthocyanidins, but only six of them are present in most foods: cyanidin, delphinidin, petunidin, peonidin, pelargonidin and malvidin. Generally speaking, anthocyanidins have a pH-dependent stability. At acidic or basic pH, the highly conjugated phenolic groups of anthocyanidins protonate and deprotonate. This causes a change in the electronic distribution, which in turn affects the absorption wavelength and the perceived colour. ATCs are formed when anthocyanidins are coupled to sugars. In red berries, the main ATCs found are anthocyanidin 3-glucosides and cyanidin-3-glucoside, which is the most common compound in most berries [156]. Berries also contain an abundance of sugars (glucose, fructose), although their calorie content is low. They contain only small amounts of fat, but are rich in dietary fibre (cellulose, hemicellulose, pectin). They also contain high levels of organic acids, such as citric acid, malic acid, tartaric acid, oxalic acid and fumaric acid, as well as trace amounts of certain minerals. **Table II** shows the nutritional values of the best-known red fruits based on USDA data.

Table II: Chemical composition of some red fruits [156].

Value/100 g	Calories (kJ)	sugars (g)	Fat (g)	Protein (g)	Vitamin C (mg)
Strawberry	136	7.68	0.3	0.67	58.8
Raspberry	196	11.94	0.65	1.20	26.2
Blueberry	240	14.49	0.33	0.74	9.7
Blackberry	180	9.61	0.49	1.39	21.0
Cranberry	190	12.20	0.13	0.39	13.3

8.3 Pharmacological properties

Because of their richness in antioxidants, notably polyphenols, and more particularly TCAs, red fruit has gained the attention of many researchers. It has been reported that TCAs have the ability to trap reactive oxygen species, inhibit lipid peroxidation and chelate metal ions, thereby reducing the risk of various diseases associated with oxidative stress **[158]**. Anthocyanin is considered a powerful nutraceutical or pharmaceutical ingredient. It has traditionally been used as a phytopharmaceutical, appetite stimulant, choleretic agent and in the treatment of many other diseases. The bioavailability of anthocyanins plays a vital role in maintaining good health and preventing disease. Low bioavailability of these pigments results in low absorption and therefore high excretion in urine and faeces, which in turn reduces the effectiveness of TCAs in scavenging free radicals. When anthocyanin is highly bioavailable, it is effective in reducing the peroxidation of cellular lipids, thereby reducing the risk of many diseases. To date, there are few reports on the bioavailability of the main TCAs for comparison. However, the major TCAs include cyanidin-3-glucoside and malvidin-3-glucoside, which have been reported to have high bioavailability [159].

Several studies have reported an association between high consumption of TFAs and a reduced risk of CVD. In fact, a meta-analysis of 6 studies found that increasing anthocyanin intake reduced the risk of cardiovascular mortality. Similar results were also reported in a meta-analysis of total CVD. In 3 cohort studies, it was found that a higher intake of TCAs resulted in a reduction of around 25% in the risk of coronary heart disease, including fatal and non-fatal myocardial infarction. Indeed, higher intakes of blueberries, strawberries and total anthocyanins were associated with a 32% lower rate of myocardial infarction, independent of established risk factors. However, in two prospective cohort studies it was found that there was no association between the intake of TCAs and the risk of stroke. Furthermore, following a high intake of TCAs, a reduction of around 8 to 10% in the risk of hypertension was observed in 5 cohort studies. Furthermore, in a cohort of over 87,000 participants examined over a period of 14 years, it was found that higher intake of TCAs resulted in a 10% lower risk of incident hypertension. The greatest reduction was observed in women aged $\leq$ 60 years. In a cross-sectional study of 1898 carefully phenotyped twins, a biomarker, vascular stiffness, was measured. In this study, a clinically relevant improvement in vascular modulation, measured using pulse wave velocity, was found and was associated with greater intake of TCAs [160]. Red fruit supplementation has been reported to help improve sports performance by reducing oxidative stress and inflammation. It seems that for these supplements to be effective, an athlete should consume the product 2 to 3 times a day at a dosage of 100 mg of anthocyanins per dose. However, further research is needed to properly assess the dose-response effects on performance gain [156]. The anti-diabetic effect of TCAs has also been widely studied. In traditional Chinese medicine, TCA-rich Cornus fruit was used to treat diabetes [159]. In a meta-analysis of data from 3 American cohorts, it was reported that high consumption of TCAs and berries was associated with a reduced risk of T2DM. Similarly, in a Polish cohort, a similar association was observed between a higher intake of TFAs and a reduced risk of T2D. In a cross-sectional study of women, a higher habitual intake of TFAs and flavones was found to improve insulin resistance. Given that obesity is positively associated with the risk of T2D, increased intake of TFAs and bilberries was associated with reduced weight gain during ageing, thus helping to reduce the risk of T2D [160]. In an animal study, it was found that obese mice fed with TFAs isolated from fruit showed a reduction in weight gain and body fat, but the differences were not always statistically significant. Purified TFAs and bilberry juice were also tested for their ability to prevent obesity by preparing a dose of 0.2 mg/mL anthocyanin in drinking water (0.49 mg/mouse/day). It was found that TCAs suppressed the rate of fat deposition. In addition, bilberry juice consumed at a rate of 2.8 mL/mouse/day (5.3 mg anthocyanin/mouse/day) did not show as effective an effect as purified TCAs in preventing fat deposition in the body. In the same context, lower serum leptin concentrations were observed following administration of purified blueberry TCAs (1 mg/mL) to obese mice for 72 days, which reduced the development of obesity [159].

In a pooled analysis of 2 US cohort studies examining nearly 150,000 people, a lower risk of Parkinson's disease was found to be associated with higher consumption of TCAs and berries. Furthermore, in a prospective analysis of 16,000 women taking part in a study of nurses' health, it was found that higher consumption of blueberries and strawberries was associated with slower rates of cognitive decline in the elderly, with an estimated delay in decline of around 2.5 years. Given that the risk of Alzheimer's disease and other dementias is linked to biomarkers of cardiovascular and metabolic risk, in particular obesity and insulin resistance in midlife, TCAs may be of great interest in preventing such diseases. In fact, higher consumption of TFAs and red fruit may be associated with a lower risk of Alzheimer's-type dementia in later life, insofar as TFAs protect against the risk of CVD and T2DM [160].

Furthermore, several studies report that extracts rich in ATC, such as bilberry, raspberry, blackcurrant and strawberry extracts, ensure the inhibition of BGN but not BGP. This variation can be explained by the different cell wall structures between BGN and BGP. The outer membrane of BGNs acts as a preventive barrier against hydrophobic compounds, but not against hydrophilic compounds such as anthocyanins. These antimicrobial activities of TCA extracts are probably the result of multiple mechanisms and synergistic actions of various phytochemical compounds in the extracts, including TCAs, weak organic acids, phenolic acids and their mixtures of different chemical forms. Thus, the antimicrobial effect of TCAs in violet, red and blue fruits should be further analysed, as they are the main bioactives in the prevention of microbial infections by several mechanisms [159].

Although the retina is protected by an active blood-brain barrier at the level of the retinal pigment epithelium, TCAs are well detected in ocular tissues. Following oral, intravenous or intraperitoneal administration of TCAs in rats and rabbits, these pigments are selectively distributed in ocular tissues. In pigs, TCAs were detected in the whole eye in a dose-dependent manner after a diet containing 0%, 1%, 2% and 4% (w/w) bilberry [160]. In fact, anthocyanin pigments are proving to be essential nutraceuticals for maintaining good vision. Berries rich in TCAs are traditionally known to be beneficial for the eyes and are often associated with night vision. In fact, oral administration of berry extract containing around 39% anthocyanins to six-week-old mice has been shown to prevent impaired photoreceptor cell function during retinal inflammation. In another study involving 132 patients with normal-tension glaucoma, two capsules of ATC (60 mg anthocyanin/capsule) were administered daily to these patients. An improvement in visual function was noted, based on the Humphrey visual field test and the minimum angle of resolution assessing best-corrected visual acuity. Certain other red fruits have a protective effect on eyesight. Supplementation with blackcurrant TCA (50mg/day) over a period of 24 months was found to increase ocular blood flow in 19 patients with open-angle glaucoma, although there were no significant effects on intraocular pressure. In addition, ATC supplementation (50mg/Kg body weight) to N-methyl-N-nitrosourea-induced retinal degeneration rats inhibited retinal degeneration and also suppressed human lens epithelial cell death under oxidative stress-inducing hydrogen peroxide (50 to 200 µg/mL extract). A reduction in lens opacity with lower levels of malonaldehyde were nevertheless associated with anthocyanin consumption [160].

8.4 Safety profile/Toxicity

With regard to anthocyanin toxicity, there are no current publications demonstrating a toxic effect reported in any of the human intervention studies. Given the low bioavailability of TCAs, the risk of toxicity from foods rich in TCAs, particularly red fruit, is minimal or non-existent. An acceptable daily intake of 2.5 mg/Kg per day has been established by the Joint FAO/WHO Expert Committee on Food Additives. This level concerns TCAs from grape skin extracts and does not apply to TCAs in general. Following a request from the European Commission to EFSA, the Scientific Panel on Food Additives and Nutrient Sources added to Food was invited to provide a scientific opinion re-evaluating the safety of ATCs. The Panel concluded that the current toxicological data base was insufficient and inadequate to establish a numerically acceptable daily intake for TFAs. Most of the toxicological data found are associated with grape skin and blackcurrant extracts and are considered unlikely to pose a safety concern by EFSA. China, being the first country to define a recommended intake for TCAs, has not defined a tolerable upper intake level. In animal studies, no toxic effects of anthocyanins (blackcurrant, blueberry and/or elderberry) were identified when administered at doses of 20mg/Kg/day in rats, 25mg/Kg/day in mice, >3g/day for 15 or 90 days in guinea pigs and rats, >2.4% of body weight in beagle dogs and 9g/Kg/day over 3 generations in rats, mice and rabbits [161].

CONCLUSION

Throughout this literature search, we have attempted to cover a variety of species that are currently widespread throughout the world. In fact, this work on superfoods has enabled us to gain a better understanding of the 'superfood' trend and to note the significant nutritional profiles of the foods studied, making them essential foodstuffs for humans. Microalgae are rich in proteins and minerals, seeds are abundant in essential fatty acids and specific bioactive compounds are present, such as monacolin K in LRR and β-glucans in LB. Some plants, notably moringa, are highly nutritious and have even been described as 'miraculous'. High levels of antioxidants have also been found in green tea (catechins) and red fruit (anthocyanosides). In addition, maca root has an exceptional nutritional profile, making it popular today as an aphrodisiac. Generally speaking, all the documents and studies found highlight the promising therapeutic properties of the components of the foodstuffs concerned, as well as other properties (colourings, preservatives, flavourings, etc.). Nevertheless, given the limitations of certain studies or questionable safety profiles, further research is required. It is also important to note that superfoods are not a substitute for medicines. For this reason, we need to be well aware of and well trained in the benefits of plants, so that we can optimise our diet and ensure a better quality of life. Faced with a growing market for plant-based remedies and a growing vegetarian trend, one avenue for future research will be to determine more precisely the recommended dosages, the adverse effects and the people targeted, in order to formalise the consumption of superfoods and perhaps one day give them a well-defined and standardised classification.

REFERENCES

1. Kim D, Ku S. Beneficial effects of monascus sp. KCCM 10093 pigments and derivatives: a mini review. Molecules. 2018;23(1):98.

2. Thomas Langenegger. Superfoods. Swiss Society of Nutrition. [Online]. 2016 [accessed January 15, 2021];(1):1-5. Available: https://www.sge-ssn.ch/media/Tabula-1-16-F-Les-superaliments.pdf

3. Superfood Info. Superfoods list of superfoods you should include in your diet [Online]. 2018 [Accessed 16 January 2021]. Available: http://superaliments.info/

4. Borowitzka MA, Gershwin ME, Belay A. Spirulina in human nutrition and health. J Appl Phycol. 2009;21(6):747.

5. Naturalforme. Spirulina, the blue algae with multiple benefits. [Online]. 2016 [Accessed 21 December 2020]. Available: https://www.naturalforme.fr/lemag/la-spiruline-bienfaits-et-proprietes/

6. Karkos PD, Leong SC, Karkos CD, Sivaji N, Assimakopoulos DA. Spirulina in clinical practice: evidence-based human applications.Evid Based Complement Alternat Med. 2011;(280):1-4.

7. Gutiérrez-Salmeán G, Fabila-Castillo L, Chamorro-Cevallos G. Nutritional and toxicological aspects of Spirulina (Arthrospira). Nutr Hosp. 2015;32(1):34-40.

8. Deng R, Chow TJ. Hypolipidemic, antioxidant and antiinflammatory activities of microalgae Spirulina.Cardiovasc Ther. 2010;28(4):33-45.

9. Mobin S, Alam F. Some promising microalgal species for commercial applications: a review. Energy Procedia. 2017;(110):510-517.

10. Belay A, Kato T, Ota Y. Spirulina (Arthrospira): potential application as an animal feed supplement. J Appl Phycol.1996;8(4):303-11.

11. Mahmoud YI, Abd El-Ghffar EA. Spirulina ameliorates aspirin-induced gastric ulcer in albino mice by alleviating oxidative stress and inflammation. Biomed Pharmacother. 2019;(109):314-21.

12. Hutadilok-Towatana N, Reanmongkol W, Satitit S, Ritthisunthorn P. A subchronic toxicity study of Spirulina platensis. Food SciTechnol Res. 2008;14(4):351-8.

13. Kunugi M, Satoh S, Ihara K, Shibata K, Yamagishi Y,Kogame K, et al. Evolution of green plants accompanied changes in light-harvesting systems. Plant Cell Physiol. 2016;57(6):1231-43.

14. Darienko T, Rad-Menéndez C, Campbell C, Pröschold T. Are there any true marine Chlorella species: molecular phylogenetic assessment and ecology of marine Chlorella-like organisms, including a description of Droopiella gen. nov.Syst Biodivers. 2019;17(8):811-29.

15. Kadalys. Chlorella. [online]. [Accessed 22 December 2020]. Available: https://kadalys.com/blogs/ingredients/chlorelle

16. Bito T, Okumura E, Fujishima M, Watanabe F. Potential of Chlorella as a dietary supplement to promote human health. Nutrients. 2020;12(9):2524.

17. Hynstova V, Sterbova D, Klejdus B, Hedbavny J, Huska D, Adam V. Separation, identification and quantification of carotenoids and chlorophylls in dietary supplements containing Chlorella vulgaris and Spirulinaplatensis using high performance thin layer chromatography. J Pharm Biomed Anal. 2018;(148):108-18.

18. Hong JW, Kim OH, Jo S-W, Kim H, Jeong MR, Park KM, et al. Biochemical composition of a korean domestic microalga Chlorella vulgaris KNUA027. Microbiol Biotechnol Lett. 2016;44(3):400-7.

19. Klamczynska B, Mooney WD. Heterotrophicmicroalgae: ascalable and sustainableprotein source. In: Nadathur SR, Wanasundara JPD, Scanlin L, editors. Sustainable protein sources [Online]. 2017 [accessed January 21, 2021]. Available: http://www.sciencedirect.com/science/article/pii/ B97801280277830002

20. Ebrahimi-Mameghani M, Sadeghi Z, Farhangi MA, Vaghef-Mehrabany E, Aliashrafi S. Glucose homeostasis, insulin resistance and inflammatory biomarkers in patients with non-alcoholic fatty liver disease: beneficial effects of supplementation with microalgae Chlorella vulgaris: a double-blind placebo-controlled randomized clinical trial. Clin Nutr. 2017;36(4):100-6.

21. Kose A, Ozen MO, Elibol M, Oncel SS. Investigation of in vitro digestibility of dietary microalga Chlorella vulgaris and cyanobacteriumSpirulinaplatensis as a nutritional supplement. 3 Biotech. 2017;7(3):170.

22. García JL, De-Vicente M, Galán B. Microalgae, old sustainable food and fashion nutraceuticals. Microb Biotechnol. 2017;10(5):1017-24.

23. Neumann U, Derwenskus F, Gille A, Louis S, Schmid-Staiger U, BrivibaK, et al. Bioavailability and safety of nutrients from the microalgae Chlorella vulgaris, Nannochloropsisoceanica and Phaeodactylumtricornutum in C57BL/6 mice. Nutrients. 2018;10(8):965.

24. Khalilnezhad A, Mahmoudian E, Mosaffa N, Anissian A, Rashidi M, Amani D. Effects of Chlorella vulgaris on tumor growth in mammary tumor-bearing Balb/c mice: discussing association of an immune-suppressed protumor microenvironment with serum IFNγ and IgG decrease and spleen IgGpotentiation. Eur J Nutr. 2018;57(3):1025-44.

25. Ozlem T, SebileA. A review on the red yeast rice (Monascus purpureus). Turk J Biotech. 2004;2(8):37-49.

26. Ma J, Li Y, Ye Q, Li J, Hua Y, Ju D, et al. Constituents of red yeast rice, a traditional Chinese food and medicine. J Agric Food Chem. 2000;48(11):5220-5.

27. Slugen D, Sturdikova M. Rosenberg M. Microbial preparation of Monascus pigments and their food applications. Bull Food ResBullet. 1997;36(3):155-169.

28. Wong HC, Koehler PE.Production and isolation of an antibiotic from Monascuspurpureus and its relationship to pigment production. J Food Sci. 1981;46(2):589-92.

29. Bakosova A, Mate D, Laciakova A, Pipova M. Utilization of Monascus purpureus in the production of foods of animal origin. Bull Vet Inst Pulawy. 2001;(45):111-116.

30. Santé magazine. Cholesterol: red yeast rice bad for the liver. [Online]. 2019 [Accessed October 10, 2020]. Available: https://www.santemagazine.fr/actualites/actualites-alimentation/cholesterol-la-levure-de-riz-rouge-mauvaise-pour-le-foie-337753

31. Chen W, He Y, Zhou Y, Shao Y, Feng Y, Li M, Chen F. Edible filamentous fungi from the species Monascus: early traditional fermentations, modern molecular biology, and future genomics. Compr Rev Food Sci Food Saf. 2015;14(5):555-67.

32. Nout MJR, Aidoo KE. Asian fungal fermented food.in: Osiewacz HD, editor. Industrial Applications [Online]. 2002 [accessed 9 October 2020]. Disponible: https://doi.org/10.1007/978-3-662-10378-4-2

33. Heber D, Yip I, Ashley JM, ElashoffDA, ElashoffRM, Go VL. Cholesterol-lowering effects of a proprietary chinese red-yeast-rice dietary supplement. Am J Clin Nutr. 1999;69(2):231-6.

34. Wang J, Lu Z, Chi J, Wang W, Su M, Kou W, et al. Multicenter clinical trial of the serum lipid-lowering effects of a Monascuspurpureus (red yeast) rice preparation from traditional Chinese medicine. Curr Ther Res. 1997;58(12):964-78.

35. Chen W, Chen R, Liu Q, He Y, He K, Ding X, et al. Orange, red, yellow: biosynthesis of azaphilone pigments in Monascus fungi. Chem Sci.

36. Vendruscolo F, Bühler RMM, De-Carvalho JC, De-Oliveira D, Moritz DE, Schmidell W, et al. Monascus: a reality on the production and application of microbial pigments. Appl Biochem Biotechnol. 2016;178(2):211-23.

37. Yang CW, Mousa SA. The effect of red yeast rice (Monascus purpureus) in dyslipidemia and other disorders. Complement Ther Med. 2012;20(6):466-74.

38. Li Y, Jiang L, Jia Z, Xin W, Yang S, Yang Q, et al. A meta-analysis of red yeast rice: an effective and relatively safe alternative approach for dyslipidemia. PLoS One. 2014;9(6):e98.

39. Han S, Jiao J, Xu J, Zimmermann D, Lucas AG, Lei G, et al. Effects of plant stanol or sterol-enriched diets on lipid profiles in patients treated with statins: systematic review and meta-analysis. Sci Rep. 2016;6(3):1337.

40 Edwards CJ, Hart DJ, Spector TD. Oral statins and increased bonemineral density in postmenopausal women. Lancet. 2000;355(9222):2218-9.

41. Wu M, Zhang WG, Liu LT. Red yeast rice prevents atherosclerosis through regulating inflammatory signaling pathways. Chin J Integr Med. 2017;23(9):689-95.

42. Jick H, Zornberg GL, Jick SS, Seshadri S, Drachman DA. Statins and the risk of dementia. Lancet. 2000;356(9242):1627-31.

43. Gheith O, Sheashaa H, Abdelsalam M, Shoeir Z, Sobh M. Efficacy and safety of Monascuspurpureus Went rice in children and young adults with secondary hyperlipidemia: a preliminary report. Eur J Intern Med. 2009;20(3):57-61.

44. EFSA panel on dietetic products, nutrition and allergies (NDA). Scientific opinion on the substantiation of health claims related to monacolin K from red yeast rice and maintenance of normal blood LDL cholesterol concentrations (ID 1648, 1700) pursuant to article 13(1) of regulation (EC) No 1924/2006. EFSA J. 2011;9(7):2304.

45. Nguyen T, Karl M, Santini A. Red Yeast Rice. Foods. 2017;6(3):19.

46. Farkouh A, Baumgärtel C. Mini-review: medication safety of red yeast rice products. Int J Gen Med. 2019;12:167-71.

47. Hatoum R, Labrie S, Fliss I. Antimicrobial and probiotic properties of yeasts: from fundamental to novel applications. Front Microbiol. 2012;(3):421.

48. ScienceDirect. Saccharomyces. [Online]. 2020 [consulted on 20 October 2020]. Available: https://www.sciencedirect.com/topics/biochemistry-genetics-and-molecular-biology/saccharomyces

49. Moyad MA. Brewer's/baker's yeast (Saccharomyces cerevisiae) and preventive medicine: part II. Urol Nurs. 2008;28(1):73-5.

50. Pérez-Torrado R, Querol A. Opportunistic strains of Saccharomyces cerevisiae: a potential risk sold in food products. Front Microbiol. 2016;(6):1522.

51. Kogan G, Pajtinka M, Babincova M, Miadokova E, Rauko P, Slamenova D, et al. Yeast cell wall polysaccharides as antioxidants and antimutagens: can they fight cancer? Neoplasma. 2008;55(5):387-93.

52. Kagertor. How to use dry yeast while brewing beer. [Online]. 2016 [Accessed 21 October 2020]. Available: https://learn.kegerator.com/dry-yeast/

53. Gray JV, Petsko GA, Johnston GC, Ringe D, Singer RA, Werner-Washburne M. "Sleeping beauty": quiescence in Saccharomyces cerevisiae. Microbiol Mol Biol Rev. 2004;68(2):187-206.

54. Liti G. The fascinating and secret wild life of the budding yeast S. cerevisiae. eLife. 2015;(4):e05835.

55. Broach JR. Nutritional Control of Growth and Development in Yeast. Genetics. 2012;192(1):73-105.

56. Dos-Santos SC, Sá-Correia I. Yeast toxicogenomics: lessons from a eukaryotic cell model and cell factory. Curr Opin Biotechnol. 2015;(33):183-91.

57. Puig-Asensio M, Padilla B, Garnacho-Montero J, Zaragoza O, Aguado JM, Zaragoza R, et al. Epidemiology and predictive factors for early and latemortality in Candida bloodstream infections: a population-based surveillance in Spain.Clin Microbiol Infect. 2014;20(4):245-54.

58. MohajeriAmiri M, Fazeli MR, Babaee T, Amini M, HayatiRoodbari N, Mousavi SB, et al. Production of vitamin D3 enriched biomass of Saccharomyces cerevisiae as a potential food supplement: evaluation and optimization of culture conditions using Plackett-Burman and response surface methodological approaches. Iran J Pharm Res. 2019;18(2):974-87.

59. Vrzhesinskaia OA, Kodentsova VM. Vitamin B1 and B2 ratio as a method of brewer's and food yeast identification. Vopr Pitan. 2004;73(3):22-5.

60. EFSA panel on dietetic products, nutrition and allergies (NDA) Scientific opinion on the safety of 'yeast beta-glucans' as a novel food ingredient. EFSA J. 2011;9(5):2137.

61. FAO/WHO. Energy and protein requirements. Report of a joint FAO/WHO/UNU Expert consultation technical report; 1985; Geneva. Switzerland: WHO; 1990.

62. Vieira EF, Carvalho J, Pinto E, Cunha S, Almeida AA, Ferreira I. Nutritive value, antioxidant activity and phenolic compounds profile of brewer's spent yeast extract. J Food Compos Anal. 2016;52:44-51.

63. Pretorius IS, Du-Toit M, Van-Rensburg P. Designer yeasts for the fermentation industry of the 21st century. Food Technol Biotechnol. 2003;41(1):3-10.

64. Parapouli M, Vasileiadis A, Afendra AS, Hatziloukas E. Saccharomyces cerevisiae and its industrial applications. AIMS Microbiol. 2020;6(1):1-31.

65. Agarbati A, Canonico L, Marini E, Zannini E, Ciani M, Comitini F. Potential probiotic yeasts sourced from natural environmental and spontaneous processed foods. Foods. 2020;9(3):287.

66. Palma ML, Zamith-Miranda D, Martins FS, Bozza FA, Nimrichter L, Montero-Lomeli M, et al. Probiotic Saccharomyces cerevisiae strains as biotherapeutic tools: is there room for improvement? Appl Microbiol Biotechnol.2015;99(16):6563-70.

67. Moré MI, Vandenplas Y. *Saccharomyces boulardii* CNCM I-745 improves intestinal enzyme function: a trophic effects review. Clin Med Insights Gastroenterol. 2018;(11):1-14.

68. Volman JJ, Ramakers JD, Plat J. Dietary modulation of immune function by beta-glucans. Physiol Behav. 2008;94(2):276-84.

69. Ryan JJ, Hanes DA, Schafer MB, Mikolai J, Zwickey H. Effect of the probiotic Saccharomyces boulardii on cholesterol and lipoprotein particles in hypercholesterolemic adults: a single-arm, open-label pilot study. J Altern Complement Med. 2015;21(5):288-93.

70. Stier H, Ebbeskotte V, Gruenwald J. Immune-modulatory effects of dietary yeast beta-1,3/1,6-D-glucan. Nutr J. 2014;13:38.

71. Hosseinzadeh P, Javanbakht MH, Mostafavi SA, Djalali M, Derakhshanian H, Hajianfar H, et al. Brewer's yeast improves glycemic indices in type 2 diabetes mellitus. Int J Prev Med. 2013;4(10):1131-8.

72. Hosseinzadeh P, Djazayry A, Mostafavi SA, Javanbakht MH, Derakhshanian H, Rahimiforoushani A, et al. Brewer's yeast improves blood pressure in type 2 diabetes mellitus. Iran J Public Health. 2013;42(6):602-9.

73. Gareis M. Ochratoxin A in brewer's yeast used as nutrient supplement. Mycotoxin Res. 2002;18(2):128-31.

74. Pancrazio G, Cunha SC, De-Pinho PG, Loureiro M, Meireles S, Ferreira IMPLVO, et al. Spent brewer's yeast extract as an ingredient in cooked hams. Meat Sci. 2016;(121):382-9.

75. Kostas K, Ana A, Avelino AO, Declan B, Sara BC, Marianne C, et al. Update of the list of QPS-recommended biological agents intentionally added to food or feed as notified to EFSA 9: suitability of taxonomic units notified to EFSA until september 2018. EFSA J. 2019;17(1):5555.

76. Pajno GB, Passalacqua G, Salpietro C, Vita D, Caminiti L, Barberio G. Looking for immunotolerance: a case of allergy to baker's yeast (Saccharomyces cerevisiae). Eur Ann Allergy Clin Immunol. 2005;37(7):271-2.

77. Di-Luzio NR, Williams DL, Mc-Namee RB, Edwards BF, Kitahama A. Comparative tumor-inhibitory and anti-bacterial activity of soluble and particulate glucan. Int J Cancer. 1979;24(6):773-9.

78. EFSA panel on dietetic products, nutrition and allergies (NDA). Scientific opinion on the safety of 'yeast beta-glucans' as a novel food ingredient. EFSA J. 2011;9(5):2137.

79. Seng P, Cerlier A, Cassagne C, Coulange M, Legré R, Stein A. Saccharomyces cerevisiae osteomyelitis in an immunocompetent baker. IDCases. 2016;(5):1-3.

80. Babícek K, Cechová I, Simon RR, Harwood M, Cox DJ. Toxicological assessment of a particulate yeast (1,3/1,6)-beta-D-glucan in rats. Food Chem Toxicol. 2007;45(9):1719-30.

81. De-Lianos R, Liopis S, Molero G, Querol A, Gil C, Fernández-Espinar MT. In vivo virulence of commercial Saccharomyces cerevisiae strains with pathogenicity-associated phenotypical traits. Int J Food Microbiol. 2011;144(3):393-9.

82. De-Lianos R, Fernández-Espinar MT, Querol A. A comparison of clinical and food Saccharomyces cerevisiae isolates on the basis of potential virulence factors. Antonie Van Leeuwenhoek. 2006;90(3):221-31.

83. Pérez-Torrado R, Liopis S, Perrone B, Gómez-Pastor R, Hube B, Querol A. Comparative genomic analysis reveals a critical role of de novo nucleotide biosynthesis for Saccharomyces cerevisiae virulence. PloS One. 2015;10(3):e0122382.

84. De-Lianos R, Liopis S, Molero G, Querol A, Gil C, Fernández-Espinar MT. In vivo virulence of commercial Saccharomyces cerevisiae strains with pathogenicity-associated phenotypical traits. Int J Food Microbiol. 2011;144(3):393-9.

85. USDA foreign agricultural service. Oilseeds: world markets and trade [Online]. 2018 [accessed January 21, 2021]. Available: https://www.fas. usda.gov/commodities/soybeans

86. Food and agriculture organization of the united nations (FAO) FAOSTAT. Food and agriculture data [Online]. 2018 [accessed 6 September 2017]. Available: http://www.fao.org/faostat/en/#home

87. Nonye B. All you need to know about soybean farming process. [Online]. 2020 [Accessed 26 December 2020]. Available: https://agric4profits.com/all-you-need-to-know-about-soybean-farming-process/

88. Song J, Liu Z, Hong H, Ma Y, Tian L, Li X, et al. Identification and validation of loci governing seed coat color by combining association mapping and bulk segregation analysis in soybean. PloS One. 2016;11(7):e0159064.

89. Lozovaya VV, Lygin AV, Ulanov AV, Nelson RL, Daydé J, Widholm JM. Effect of temperature and soil moisture status during seed development on soybean seed isoflavone concentration and composition. Crop Sci. 2005;45(5):1934-40.

90. Huang H, Krishnan HB, Pham Q, Yu LL, Wang TTY. Soy and gut microbiota: interaction and implication for human health. J Agric Food Chem. 2016;64(46):8695-709.

91. Kumar P, Chatli MK, Mehta N, Singh P, Malav OP, Verma AK. Meat analogues: health promising sustainable meat substitutes. Crit Rev Food Sci Nutr. 2017;57(5):923-32.

92. Keinan-Boker L, Peeters PHM, Mulligan AA, Navarro C, Slimani N, Mattisson I, et al. Soy product consumption in 10 European countries: the European Prospective Investigation into Cancer and Nutrition (EPIC) study. Public Health Nutr. 2002;5(6B):1217-26.

93. Espinosa-Martos I, Rupérez P. Soybean oligosaccharides: potential as new ingredients in functional food. Nutr Hosp. 2006;21(1):92-6.

94. Zaheer K, Humayoun Akhtar M. An updated review of dietary isoflavones: nutrition, processing, bioavailability and impacts on human health. Crit Rev Food Sci Nutr. 2017;57(6):1280-93.

95. Amigo-Benavent M, Silván JM, Moreno FJ, Villamiel M, Del-Castillo MD. Protein quality, antigenicity, and antioxidant activity of soy-based foodstuffs. J Agric Food Chem. 2008;56(15):6498-505.

96. Rizzo G, Baroni L. Soy, soy foods and their role in vegetarian diets. Nutrients. 2018;10(1):43.

97. Barnes S, Boersma B, Patel R, Kirk M, Darley-Usmar VM, Kim H, et al. Isoflavonoids and chronic disease: mechanisms of action. Bio Factors Oxf Engl. 2000;12(1-4):209-15.

98. Ko KP. Isoflavones: chemistry, analysis, functions and effects on health and cancer. Asian Pac J Cancer Prev. 2014;15(17):7001-10.

99. Mazur WM, Duke JA, Wähälä K, Rasku S, Adlercreutz H. Isoflavonoids and lignans in legumes: nutritional and health aspects in humans. J Nutr Biochem. 1998;9(4):193-200.

100. Howitz KT, Sinclair DA. Xenohormesis: sensing the chemical cues of other species. Cell. 2008;133(3):387-91.

101. Piotrowska E, Jakóbkiewicz-Banecka J, Wegrzyn G. Different amounts of isoflavones in various commercially available soy extracts in the light of gene expression-targeted isoflavone therapy. Phytother Res.
2010;24 (1):109-13.

102. Russo M, Russo GL, Daglia M, Kasi PD, Ravi S, Nabavi SF, et al. Understanding genistein in cancer: the "good" and the "bad" effects: a review. Food Chem. 2016;196:589-600.

103. Grosso G, Bella F, Godos J, Sciacca S, Del Rio D, Ray S, et al. Possible role of diet in cancer: systematic review and multiple meta-

analyses of dietary patterns, lifestyle factors, and cancer risk. Nutr Rev. 2017;75(6):405-19.

104. Mejía W, Córdoba D, Durán P, Chacón Y, Rosselli D. Effect of daily exposure to an isolated soy protein supplement on body composition, energy and macronutrient intake, bone formation markers, and lipid profile in children in Colombia. J Diet. 2019;16(1):1-13.

105. Duitama SM, Zurita J, Cordoba D, Duran P, Ilag L, Mejia W. Soy protein supplement intake for 12 months has no effect on sexual maturation and may improve nutritional status in pre-pubertal children. J Paediatr Child Health. 2018;54(9):997-1004.

106. Touillaud M, Gelot A, Mesrine S, Bennetau-Pelissero C, Clavel-Chapelon F, Arveux P, et al. Use of dietary supplements containing soy isoflavones and breast cancer risk among women aged >50 y: a prospective study. Am J Clin Nutr. 2019;109(3):597-605.

107. De-Falco B, Amato M, Lanzotti V. Chia seeds products: an overview. Phytochem Rev. 2017;(16):745-760.

108. Mohd-Ali N, Yeap SK, Ho WY, Beh BK, Tan SW, Tan SG. The promising future of chia, Salvia hispanica L. J Biomed Biotechnol. 2012;(2012):171956.

109. Das A. Advances in Chia seed research. Adv Biotechnol Microbiol. 2018;(5):5-7.

110. Campos BE, Dias-Ruivo T, Da-Silva-Scapim MR, Madrona GS, De-C-Bergamasco R. Optimization of the mucilage extraction process from chia seeds and application in ice cream as a stabilizer and emulsifier. LWT Food Sci Technol. 2016;65:874-83.

111. Ullah R, Nadeem M, Khalique A, Imran M, Mehmood S, Javid A, et al. Nutritional and therapeutic perspectives of Chia (Salvia hispanica L.): a review. J Food Sci Technol. 2016;53(4):1750-8.

112. Grancieri M, Martino HSD, Gonzalez-De-Mejia E. Chia seed (Salvia hispanica L.) as a source of proteins and bioactive peptides with health benefits: a review. Compr Rev Food Sci Food Saf. 2019;18(2):480-499.

113. Segura-Campos MR, Ciau-Solís N, Rosado-Rubio G, Chel-Guerrero L, Betancur-Ancona D. Chemical and functional properties of chia seed (Salvia hispanica L.) gum. Intern J Food Sci. 2014;(2014):e241053.

114 Hentry HS, Mittleman M, Mc-Crohan PR. Introduccion de la chia y la goma de tragacanto en los EstadosUnidos. In: Janick OJ, Simon JE, editors. Advances in New Cosechas. Portland OH: Prensa de la Madera; 1990. p. 252-256.

115. Knez-Hrnčič M, Cör D, Knez Ž. Subcritical extraction of oil from black and white chia seeds with n-propane and comparison with conventional techniques. J Supercrit Fluids. 2018;140:182-7.

116. Cahill JP. Ethnobotany of chia,Salvia hispanica L. (Lamiaceae). Econ Bot. 2003;(57):604-618.

117. Silva C, Garcia V A S, Zanette C M. Chia (Salvia hispanica L.) oil extraction using different organic solvents: oil yield, fatty acids profile and technological analysis of defatted meal. Int Food Res J. 2016;23(3):998-1004.

118. Muñoz LA, Cobos A, Diaz O, Aguilera JM. Chia seeds: microstructure, mucilage extraction and hydration. J Food Eng. 2012;108(1):216-24.

119. Kulczyński B, Kobus-Cisowska J, Taczanowski M, Kmiecik D, Gramza-Michałowska A. The chemical composition and nutritional

value of chia seeds-current state of knowledge. Nutrients. 2019;11(6):1242.

120. Beltrán-Orozco MC, Romero MR. Chía, alimentomilenario. Rev Ind Aliment. 2003;(5):20-29.

121 Knez-Hrnčič M, Ivanovski M, Cör D, Knez Ž. Chia seeds (Salvia Hispanica L.): an overview, phytochemical profile, isolation methods, and application. Molecules. 2019;25(1):11.

122. Julio LM, Ixtaina VY, Fernández MA, Sánchez RMT, Wagner JR, Nolasco SM, et al. Chia seed oil-in-water emulsions as potential delivery systems of ω-3 fatty acids. J Food Eng. 2015;162:48-55.

123. Nadeem M, Ajmal M, Rahman F, Ayaz M. Analytical characterization of butter oil enriched with omega-3 and 6 fatty acids through chia (Salvia hispanica L.) seed oil. Pak J Anal Environ Chem. 2015;16(2):68-71.

124 Repo-Carrasco-Valencia R, Hellström JK, Pihlava J-M, Mattila PH. Flavonoids and other phenolic compounds in Andean indigenous grains: Quinoa (Chenopodium quinoa), kañiwa (Chenopodiumpallidicaule) and kiwicha (Amaranthuscaudatus). Food Chem. 2010;120(1):128-33.

125 Noshe AS, Al-Bayyar AH. Effect of extraction method of chia seeds oil on its content of fatty acids and antioxidants. Int Res J Eng Tech. 2017;4(10):545-551.

126. Da-Luz JMR, Nunes MD, Paes SA, Torres DP, De-Cássia-Soares, Da-Silva M, Kasuya MCM. Lignocellulolytic enzyme production of pleurotusostreatus growth in agroindustrial wastes. Braz J Microbiol Publ B. 2012;43(4):1508-15.

127. Rahman MJ, De-Camargo AC, Shahidi F. Phenolic and polyphenolic profiles of chia seeds and their in vitro biological activities. J Funct Foods. 2017;35:622-34.

128. Alcântara MA, De-Lima-Brito-Polari I, De-Albuquerque-Meireles BRL, De Lima AEA, Da-Silva-Junior JC, De-Andrade-Vieira É, et al. Effect of the solvent composition on the profile of phenolic compounds extracted from chia seeds. Food Chem. 2019;275:489-96.

129. Guindani C, Podestá R, Block JM, Rossi MJ, Mezzomo N, Ferreira SRS. Valorization of chia (Salvia hispanica) seed cake by means of supercritical fluid extraction. J Supercrit Fluids. 2016;112:67-75.

130 Reyes-Caudillo E, Tecante A, Valdivia-López MA. Dietary fibre content and antioxidant activity of phenolic compounds present in Mexican chia (Salvia hispanica L.) seeds. Food Chem. 2008;107(2):656-63.

131. Sargi SC, Silva BC, Santos HMC, Montanher PF, Boeing JS, Santos Júnior OO, et al. Antioxidant capacity and chemical composition in seeds rich in omega-3: chia, flax, and perilla. Food Sci Technol. 2013;33(3):541-8.

132. Brglez-Mojzer E, Knez-Hrnčič M, Škerget M, Knez Ž, Bren U. Polyphenols: extraction methods, antioxidative action, bioavailability and anticarcinogenic effects. Molecules. 2016;21(7):901.

133. De-Falco B, Fiore A, Rossi R, Amato M, Lanzotti V. Metabolomics driven analysis by UAEGC-MS and antioxidant activity of chia (Salvia hispanica L.) commercial and mutant seeds. Food Chem. 2018;254:137-43.

134. Food law consultants (The chia company). Request for scientific evaluation of substantial equivalence application for the approval of

chia seeds (Salvia hispanica L.) from the chia company for use in bread [Online]. 2010 [Accessed 23 January 2021]. Available: https://acnfp.food.gov.uk/sites/default/files/mnt/drupal_data/sources /files/multimedia/pdfs/thechiacompany.pdf

135. Borneo R, Aguirre A, León AE. Chia (Salvia hispanica L) gel can be used as egg or oil replacer in cake formulations. J Am Diet Assoc. 2010;110(6):946-9.

136. Ayerza JR, Coates W. Chia: rediscovering a forgotten crop of the Aztecs. USA: The university of Arizona press; 2005.

137. Fernandez I, Vidueiros S, Ayerza R, Coates W, Pallaro A. Impact of chia (Salvia hispanica L.) on the immune system: preliminary study. PNS. 2008;67(1):e12.

138. Turck D, Castenmiller J, De-Henauw S, Hirsch-Ernst KI, Kearney J, Maciuk A, et al. Safety of chia seeds (Salvia hispanica L.) as a novel food for extended uses pursuant to Regulation (EU) 2015/2283. EFSA J. 2019;17(4):e05657.

139. Meireles D, Gomes J, Lopes L, Hinzmann M, Machado J. A review of properties, nutritional and pharmaceutical applications of Moringaoleifera: integrative approach on conventional and traditional Asian medicine. Adv Tradit Med. 2020;1-21.

140 Stohs SJ, Hartman MJ. Review of the safety and efficacy of Moringaoleifera. Phytother Res. 2015;29(6):796-804.

141. indiamart. Moringa oleifera leaves, packaging size: 1 Kg, packaging type: Pouch. [Online]. 2012 [Accessed 30 December 2020]. Available: https://www.indiamart.com/proddetail/moringa-oleifera-leaves-10452962612 .html

142. Su B, Chen X. Current status and potential of Moringaoleifera leaf as an alternative protein source for animal feeds. Front Vet Sci. 2020;(7):53.

143. Abdull-Razis AF, Ibrahim MD, Kntayya SB. Health benefits of Moringaoleifera. AsianPac J Cancer Prev. 2014;15(20):8571-6.

144. Vergara-Jimenez M, Almatrafi MM, Fernandez ML. Bioactive components in Moringaoleifera leaves protect against chronic disease. Antioxidants. 2017;6(4):91.

145. Bhattacharya A, Tiwari P, Sahu PK, Kumar S. A review of the phytochemical and pharmacological characteristics of Moringa oleifera. J Pharm Bioallied Sci. 2018;10(4):181-91.

146. Kou X, Li B, Olayanju JB, Drake JM, Chen N. Nutraceutical or pharmacological potential of Moringaoleifera Lam. Nutrients. 2018;10(3):343.

147. Abd Rani NZ, Husain K, Kumolosasi E. Moringa Genus: a review of phytochemistry and pharmacology. Front Pharmacol. 2018;(9):108.

148. Thorne Research. Green tea.Altern Med Rev. 2000;5(4):372-5.

149. Prasanth MI, Sivamaruthi BS, Chaiyasut C, Tencomnao T. A review of the role of green tea (Camellia sinensis) in antiphotoaging, stress resistance, neuroprotection, and autophagy. Nutrients. 2019;11(2):474.

150 Effinov, individualised micronutrition. Why is green tea good for you? [Online]. 2019 [Accessed 16 January 2021]. Available: https://www.effinov-nutrition.fr/blog/pourquoi-le-the-vert-est-bon-pour-la-sante-n50

151. Chacko SM, Thambi PT, Kuttan R, Nishigaki I. Beneficial effects of green tea: a literature review. Chin Med. 2010;(5):13.

152. Musial C, Kuban-Jankowska A, Gorska-Ponikowska M. Beneficial properties of green tea catechins. Int J Mol Sci. 2020;21(5):1744.

153. Gonzales GF. Ethnobiology and ethnopharmacology of lepidium meyenii (Maca), a plant from the peruvian highlands. Evid-Based Complement Altern Med. 2012;(2012):e193496.

154. Beharry S, Heinrich M. Is the hype around the reproductive health claims of maca (Lepidium meyenii Walp.) justified? J Ethnopharmacol. 2018;(211):126-70.

155. Gonzales GF, Gasco M, Lozada I. Role of maca (Lepidiummeyenii) consumption on serum interleukin-6 levels and health status in populations living in the peruvian central andes over 4000 m of altitude. Plant Foods Hum Nutr. 2013;68(4):347-51.

156. Hidalgo G-I, Almajano MP. Red fruits: extraction of antioxidants, phenolic content, and radical scavenging determination: a review. Antioxidants. 2017;6(1):7.

157. Elodie H. 7 foods for beautiful skin. [Online]. 2015 [Accessed 15 January 2021]. Available: https://www.pleinevie.fr/sante/nutrition/7-aliments-pour-une-belle-peau-12196

158. Bloedon TK, Braithwaite RE, Carson IA, Klimis-Zacas D, Lehnhard RA. Impact of anthocyanin-rich whole fruit consumption on exercise-induced oxidative stress and inflammation: a systematic review and meta-analysis. Nutr Rev. 2019;77(9):630-45.

159. Khoo HE, Azlan A, Tang ST, Lim SM. Anthocyanidins and anthocyanins: colored pigments as food, pharmaceutical ingredients, and the potential health benefits. Food Nutr Res. 2017;61(1):e1361779.

160 Kalt W, Cassidy A, Howard LR, Krikorian R, Stull AJ, Tremblay F, et al. Recent research on the health benefits of blueberries and their anthocyanins. Adv Nutr. 2020;11(2):224-36.

161. Wallace TC, Giusti MM. Anthocyanins1. Adv Nutr. 2015;6(5):620-2.

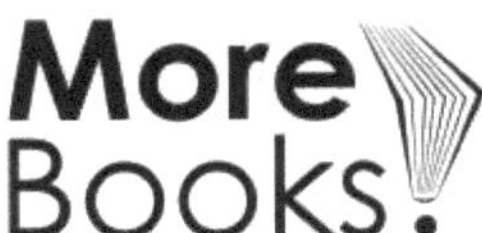
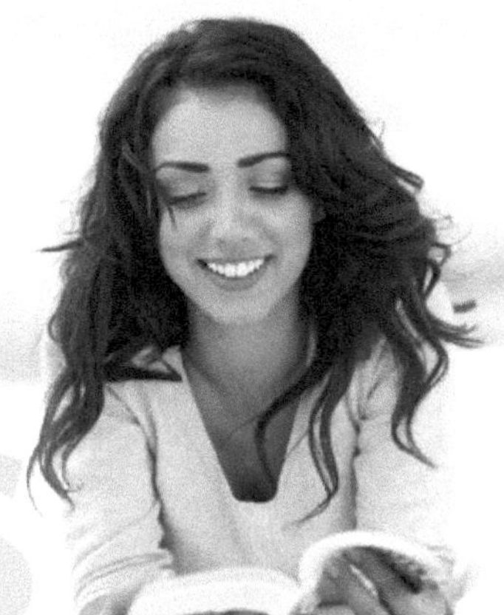

I want morebooks!

Buy your books fast and straightforward online - at one of world's fastest growing online book stores! Environmentally sound due to Print-on-Demand technologies.

Buy your books online at
www.morebooks.shop

Kaufen Sie Ihre Bücher schnell und unkompliziert online – auf einer der am schnellsten wachsenden Buchhandelsplattformen weltweit! Dank Print-On-Demand umwelt- und ressourcenschonend produziert.

Bücher schneller online kaufen
www.morebooks.shop

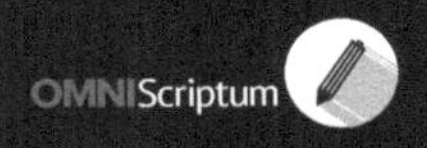

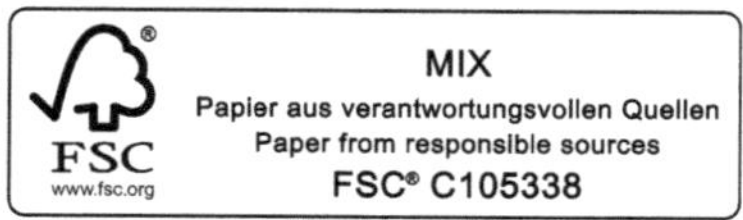

Printed by Books on Demand GmbH, Norderstedt / Germany